Atkins Diet for Busy Women

Look and Feel Better by Eating Satisfying Foods You Really Enjoy

Nathalie Seaton

declared or implied. Readers acknowledge that the author is not engaging in the rendering of legal, financial, medical or professional advice. The content within this book has been derived from various sources. Please consult a licensed professional before attempting any techniques outlined in this book.

By reading this document, the reader agrees that under no circumstances is the author responsible for any losses, direct or indirect, which are incurred as a result of the use of the information contained within this document, including, but not limited to, — errors, omissions, or inaccuracies.

Table of Contents

Chapter 11: Low-Carb Dinner Recipes _____*186*

Chapter 12: Low-Carb Recipes for the Sweet Tooth _____*207*

Chapter 13: Delicious Low-Carb Smoothies and Beverages _____*224*

SPECIAL BONUS!

Want This Bonus book for FREE?

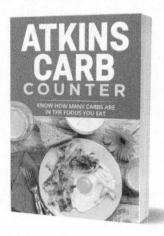

Get <u>FREE</u> unlimited access to it and all of my new books by joining the Fan Base!

SCAN W/ YOUR CAMERA TO JOIN!

Introduction

The Atkins Diet has been tried and tested for decades, with proven results. Although it is a popular celebrity diet, it was designed to suit the needs and budget of everyone. The Atkins Diet was created to help people eat everyday whole foods more beneficially. You will probably already have a lot of the approved diet foods in your pantry because you eat normal everyday foods on the Atkins Diet. Because you eat regular foods that you can buy at any grocery store, the diet is easily adapted to fit into your lifestyle. You will look and feel better while still eating the satisfying foods you really enjoy.

Dieting the Atkins way means only having to make some adjustments to your eating habits, and not your entire way of life. Most other diets make you slash your portion size, which leaves you feeling hungry and more inclined to cheat or give up. Although the Atkins Diet recommends portion control, it is in the sense that you eat until you're full and don't overeat or exceed your recommended daily carbohydrate allowance.

On the Atkins Diet, there is no calorie counting, on again or off again days, or fasting intervals. You eat three square meals a day with room for two light snacks in between. You won't feel hungry during the day. Because you are limiting your carb intake and not overeating, your body burns fat as its fuel source, thus leaving you feeling more alive, energized, and alert. You will also look amazing and have a lot more confidence.

There are many benefits to living the Atkins way. One of which ensures that those extra pounds you lose stay off for good. An Atkins lifestyle will also improve the quality of your life and health. Once you have been on the diet for a couple of weeks, you will realize just how easy it is to slip into the Atkins way of life.

As the Atkins Diet means making healthier choices from the foods you love, if you have family, there is no need to make two separate meals each mealtime. Your family can also enjoy and benefit from the delicious healthy meals you make on this diet.

Women face many body change challenges throughout their life. We go through puberty, pregnancy, menopause, and the many other growing pains in between. While all this is happening, we still have to deal with our everyday lives. What is so great about the Atkins Diet is that it can be adjusted and adapted to fit into our busy lifestyles! We don't have to make drastic changes to fit our lifestyle into it. No matter if you are pregnant, breastfeeding, raising children, or menopausal, the Atkins Diet can work for you.

There is one thing that can put a person off the Atkins Diet, especially a person with an already hectic life. At first glance, the diet appears a little complex and not everyone has the time to browse through websites and books with conflicting information. I know this firsthand from when I started on the Atkins diet some years ago as a busy woman with a family, an executive job, and fast heading towards middle age. There were several times I wanted to quit because I did not have the time to dig for the information I needed, especially in the first two weeks of the diet when your body is adjusting to the limited carb intake and you are trying to overcome your cravings.

I have had a lot of success on the Atkins Diet and feel that my family has also benefited from my healthier and carb-conscious choices. I started having children late in life and struggled to lose a lot of the weight I had gained with my firstborn. That is when I started the Atkins Diet. To be honest, it was a battle for me in the beginning and it did not need to be; this inspired me to write this book.

I have written *Atkins Diet for Busy Women* to help

you save time getting started on the Atkins Diet plan. The book breaks the Atkins Diet into easy to follow sections. There is a comprehensive list of approved foods and their net carb value per portion size per phase. There is also a comprehensive list of foods to avoid.

To make your meal planning easier, I have included a seven-day meal plan for Phase 1 and Phase 2 to get you started. There are a few exercise ideas to add to the benefits of your healthier lifestyle along with what common mistakes to avoid when getting started and step-by-step delicious low-carb recipes to try. By the end of this book, you will know exactly how the Atkins Diet works and be well on your way to achieving your weight loss goals.

Chapter 1: The Atkins Diet

Dr. Robert Atkins was a cardiologist who introduced the Atkins diet in the 1960s. He developed this diet because of his growing concerns for the increase of the overweight and obese.

If you eat more carbohydrates than your body can use, it will store the excess carbs as fat. This means you are at greater risk of gaining weight. Carrying excess weight may increase a person's risk of developing diseases such as diabetes or heart disease.

The Atkins Diet plan limits the number of carbohydrates in a diet according to a person's needs while increasing proteins and fats. It is not a diet that needs you to count calories, and it does not limit portion sizes. However, you need to be aware of the number of carbohydrates you are eating per day. Most foods you buy at the store these days come with a nutritional label on it. This makes it easy to keep track of each food item's carbohydrate value.

When the Atkins Diet first came out, they nicknamed it the "steak and eggs diet" because the diet allowed fried eggs and fatty meat cuts. Because of Dr. Atkins' fresh approach to losing weight, his diet plan was, at first, highly criticized. Over the years, thousands of people have successfully lost weight on his diet plan. Not only have they lost weight, but by adopting the Atkin's way of eating as a lifestyle, they have kept the weight off.

Since Dr. Atkins introduced the diet plan, it has been adapted and refined to move with the times and health trends over the decades. In the modern-day era, the diet can adapt to suit any lifestyle, including vegetarians and vegans.

How the Atkins Diet Works

Unlike a lot of other diet plans, the Atkins Diet does not require calorie counting, or on again off again days, and there are no restrictive portion controls. A regular diet that counts calories may still not sufficiently control or limit carbs in the diet. This can cause problems such as feeling flat, tired, and moody because carbs affect blood sugar.

The Atkins Diet requires a person to keep tight control of the carbohydrates they consume during the day. Your body will no longer burn sugar; instead, it will burn fat during the day if you limit the number of carbs you eat. As a result, you will feel more awake, energized, and alert while shedding pounds.

There are three different Atkins plans to choose from; the plan you choose will depend on your weight loss or lifestyle goals. The three Atkins diet plans are:

Atkins 20 Diet Plan

This is the original Atkins diet plan and the most popular one to start with.

- The diet plan is broken into four different phases (Phase 1 to Phase 4), and each phase has a set amount of carbs you can eat per day. As you reach your goal weight and progress to the next phase, you can slowly increase the amount and types of carbs you eat per day.
- In Phase 1, you will eat 20 to 25 grams of carbs per day.
- It is a diet plan for anyone who has more than 40 pounds to lose.
- It is also a good diet for anyone who is either pre-diabetic or diabetic.
- It is for someone who wants to maintain their weight and adapt the diet as a lifestyle. People looking to maintain their weight usually start at Phase 3 or 4 of this plan.

Atkins 40 Diet Plan

This is an Atkins diet plan that has a little more flexibility with the type of carbs you eat and the amount you eat per day.

- On this plan, you will start with 40 grams of carbs per day.
- Your carb intake will increase by 10 grams when you reach your goal weight.
- This diet is ideal for anyone who has fewer than 40 pounds to lose.
- It is ideal for women who are pregnant or breastfeeding (under the strict guidance of a doctor or health care advisor).
- This Atkins diet plan gives you a larger selection of foods you can eat from the start.

Atkins 100 Diet Plan

This plan is for those who are wanting to make the Atkins Diet an everyday part of their healthy eating plans.

- On this plan, you will start with 100 grams of carbs per day.

- Your carb intake and portion controls stay the same.
- This diet is ideal for anyone who wants to maintain their current weight and eat healthier.
- Under the strict guidance of a doctor or health care provider, it can be used by women who are pregnant or breastfeeding.
- This Atkins diet plan allows you the freedom to choose the foods that you want to eat within the given carb limitations.

Please note that these three plans are as they appear on the atkins.com website at the time this book was printed. Some global Atkins websites do not offer or reference these three plans. You may find that these global sites still use the Atkins Diet Phase 1 through 4 for weight loss, weight control maintenance, and lifestyle plans.

Remember to always check with a doctor before starting any new weight loss or lifestyle plans. This is especially important if you have an existing health issue or are pregnant.

What Are the Benefits of the Atkins Diet?

There are many reasons for eating a low-carbohydrate diet. Here are some major benefits:

- Your body burns fat instead of carbohydrates for energy, resulting in the loss of excess body fat.
- Cravings of carbohydrate-rich food eventually stop, breaking the cycle of overeating because of carb highs and lows.
- When the cravings stop, you don't feel hungry all the time.
- The Atkins Diet promotes an improved level of HDL (the good cholesterol your body needs).
- You feel more alert as your concentration improves and blood-sugar stabilizes.
- Stable blood sugar levels also improve upon a person's moods, and you will have fewer mood swings.

- You will feel less bloated within a week or two from starting a low-carb diet. This is because carbs encourage the body to retain water.
- As there is no counting calories or a set food plan; you are more likely to find something you can eat on a menu at a restaurant.
- Overall, you will feel more energetic, you will not feel so tired all the time, and you will look and feel great about yourself.

Atkins Results & Inspirational Success Stories

Please note that the names in the stories have been changed.

Pam — 25 years old from California — Lost 20 pounds

Pam had been overweight since going through puberty in her late teens. Through ups and downs in her personal life and having a baby halfway through college, her weight increased. As her weight increased, Pam became more and more insecure and started to grow to dislike herself. The more she disliked her body, the more she would comfort herself with high-carb and sugar-filled foods. Until one day her husband started to follow the Atkins Diet plan. Intrigued by how well her husband was eating and what he could eat, Pam decided to give it a go. That was three years ago. Not only did Pam manage to lose all that weight, but by making some changes to her eating habit and exercising, she has also managed to keep the weight off. She is more confident, has more energy, and looks absolutely stunning. Pam is a busy mom of three, who has easily managed to adapt the Atkins Lifestyle to fit into her way of life.

Desire — 49 years old from Boston — Lost 18 pounds

Up until Desire was 39 years old, she had always been super health-conscious and fit. She had her first baby at the age of 39. She kept up her vigorous exercise routine well into her fourth trimester of pregnancy. During the last month of her pregnancy, her body seemed to pop out and she gained quite a bit of weight. Once her baby was born, the weight kept piling. As a busy new mother, career woman, and wife, she hardly had time to breathe, let alone think about her eating habits. When her son was five years old, he asked her if she had another baby in her belly because it was so big. That is when Desire decided it was time to find a way to lose weight. She needed a diet that was more than an eating plan and one that she could easily fit around her entire family. That is

21

when she found the Atkins Diet. Desire lost 18 pounds five years ago, and losing those pounds changed her life for the better. Living the Atkins Lifestyle, Desire has managed to keep those pounds at bay. She still enjoys the foods she loves, and by making a few changes for each member of her family to the diet, she keeps her family eating healthy as well.

Jackie — 55 years old from New York — Lost 65 pounds

Jackie struggled to lose weight as she juggled a high-stress job, a messy divorce, and getting used to an empty nest. After her children left home to study or move on with their own lives, Jackie threw herself into her work to fill the void. As she no longer had anyone to cook for, fast foods, TV dinners, or a snack bar became her everyday meals. Being over 50, Jackie was also going through menopause, which added to the weight gain effects of her unhealthy eating habits. After many failed attempts at fad diets, Jackie gave up with her weight until her daughter got engaged to be married. It was not long after that, that Jackie found out she was pre-diabetic and was warned to lose weight. Her health scare and her daughter's upcoming marriage were Jackie's wake-up call. A friend of hers introduced her to the Atkins Diet, and with the support of her family and friends,

Jackie lost 65 pounds. That was three years ago and to date Jackie has kept the weight off, she now lives a healthy Atkins Lifestyle and is engaged to be married once again. Her health has improved, she feels more energized and alive than she ever felt before going on the Atkins Diet.

Chapter 2: Where to Begin

Deciding to change your eating habits to improve your health is the first big step to a healthier lifestyle. Choosing the correct diet is the second step in starting a diet. Most people skip the next few steps and dive right into their diets. There is nothing wrong with being eager to get your diet started and the path to shedding those extra pounds or being healthy. In fact, being eager and excited over changing your eating habits is a good start.

A successful diet means self-preparation and organization. You may know why you need to diet, how you are going to diet, and the foods to eat. But that may not prepare you for the impact it will have on you or your life. Being eager to start the diet will not keep you motivated for too long if you are not fully prepared. This chapter will help you better prepare yourself for getting started on your Atkins Diet journey. It will help you set realistic goals, find challenges you may face, help you understand supplements, and more.

Are There Health Risks?

As with any diet, there are always health risks. This is especially true if you have preexisting health conditions and/or are pregnant, menopausal, or of an advanced age.

The beginning of the Atkins Diet, Phase 1, drastically cuts a person's carb intake and can cause some side effects. Some of the most common side effects experienced on the Atkins Diet are:

- Constipation
- Dizziness
- Fatigue
- Headache
- Weakness

Should any of the symptoms persist or you become concerned, seek immediate medical advice.

If you can stick to the Atkins Diet and get over the first few weeks, the diet can have some positive effects on your health. It may also improve on some serious health conditions which include:

- Cardiovascular disease
- Diabetes
- Improve blood cholesterol
- High blood pressure
- Metabolic syndrome

Adjusting the Atkins Diet During Pregnancy, Breast Feeding, Post Menopause

In pregnancy, and under the careful guidance of your doctor, you can maintain a healthy weight. Any extra pounds you may have gained will be a lot easier to shed when you can eat normally again.

Women who are heading for or going through menopause have to take extra care with what foods they eat. You also have to consider the hormone fluctuations, lack of sleep as your sleep patterns change, loss of muscle mass, and an increase in insulin resistance. Low-carb diets, such as the Atkins Diet, have been shown to be far more effective for weight loss at this time of a woman's life, especially for getting rid of belly fat (Gardner et al., 2007).

As there are risks to any diet, this risk can increase if a woman is pregnant, breastfeeding, or post-menopausal. The Atkins websites have some documentation on this, but it is best to seek the advice of a doctor or nutritionist. Trained specialists will adjust and adapt the Atkins diet to suit your individual needs. When you are pregnant, there are certain foods you need to avoid, and this is the same if you are breastfeeding. Although there are general foods to avoid like shellfish, coffee, alcohol, etc., your pregnancy may require extra nutrients or specific dietary requirements.

When a woman is premenopausal, you may require extra nutrients and supplements. These will need to be expertly fit into your diet to ensure proper weight loss and be beneficial to your health. Once again, although following the diet as it is will still be beneficial, to get the most from the Atkins Diet it is best to seek a licensed professional's advice.

Am I Ready to Change My Lifestyle?

One of the big questions you should ask yourself before you jump in and begin dieting is *"Am I ready to change my lifestyle?"* Because that is what you are doing: you are making a change to your lifestyle. One of the big reasons most diets fail is because people see them as a quick fix to losing weight.

The sad reality is that a lot of these fad diets are just a way to shed a few pounds fast. A lot of these diets do offer quick weight loss, but as with everything that seems too good to be true, these diets don't work. They may seem like they are working at first. You may even see results quite fast. But for how long will you keep that weight off? What cost to your health, your well-being, and your pocket did you have to pay?

If you are reading this book, then you have decided it is time to make a more drastic change to your eating habits. With the success rate of the Atkins diet, you have made the right choice. But deciding it is time for a change and finding the right diet is only part of the process of getting ready for a lifestyle change. Another part of the dieting process is accepting that this is not just a diet. It is a lifestyle; you are going to have to make some changes. But with Atkins, the changes are not that drastic.

You need to ask yourself the following questions:

- Why am I wanting to diet?
- What am I trying to accomplish?
- Do I want to lose weight for a special occasion?
- Do I want to lose the extra pounds I have gained recently or over the years?
- Do I want to get healthy?
- Do I want to make sure the pounds I lose stay off for good?
- Am I ready to change my eating habits and commit to a healthier lifestyle?

The Atkins Diet is about learning to eat the foods you love the right way. I am not going to lie because there are some foods you will have to do away with. But the good news is there are always healthier alternatives to substitute the foods with.

You just have to commit to making the changes and give them a try. One of the best things about the Atkins diet is that you don't have to turn your life upside down. You choose the foods you want to eat from the acceptable foods list. For the first two weeks, you do have a limited selection, but it is quite a large list of foods on that list.

The diet does not end after the first two weeks. You progress onto the next phase of the diet, which introduces an even wider variety of food choices. As you progress to the maintenance and lifestyle phase, you realize how simple eating healthy actually is. That a few simple changes in what you eat and how you eat it can make a huge difference to your weight and overall health.

For a diet to be successful, you need to commit to it for a lifetime. Otherwise, your weight and health will most likely continue to yo-yo back and forth. Do you really want to put all this effort into losing weight and getting healthy, only to fall back into bad habits? Looking at a diet as something you have to do for a certain length of time is why most people land right back where they started.

Now, ask yourself again, are you ready to commit to a lifestyle change?

Think of it as cleaning out your closet and everything you get rid of, must go for good. You are going to keep all the basics and your favorites, but you are going to shake things up a little and add a few new bits. By the time you have finished your first two weeks on the diet, your body will have already started to adjust to the new routine. After four weeks, you will find that even the way you grocery shop will have changed.

So, if you are ready for a wardrobe change, then it is time to take the next step.

What Are My Goals?

There are no quick fixes or magic potions you can take that will make the pounds dissolve or magically transform you. Now that you are ready to make the change for a healthier, slimmer you, you don't want to stumble at your first hurdle. That first hurdle for most people looking to lose weight is setting realistic goals.

Losing weight too quickly may seem like a good thing but it is not. Not only is it mostly water your body loses, but it is not very good for your health. To burn fat, you need to have a healthy balance of carbohydrates in your body. Not too much that your body will store the excess as fat, but not too little that your body has no energy reserves either.

If you do lose weight too quickly, your body will quickly reach a plateau where your weight loss will slow down or stop altogether. This also becomes a turning point for some people and they just throw in the towel, then revert to their old habits. Then there is the part where you may look good having shed those pounds but you probably don't feel that great. To get there more than likely took a lot out of you physically, mentally, and emotionally.

Stick to the wise words of the tortoise in the story about the tortoise and the hare, *"Slow and steady wins the race."* A healthy weekly weight loss should be no more than one to two pounds. If you are exercising, you will need to set goals and an achievable routine to accommodate your fitness plan. As with weight loss, set steady achievable goals for yourself that are not going to wear you out and leave you aching.

If you have any pre-existing conditions, concerns, or need a bit of advice, speak to a healthcare professional, nutritionist, or dietician. They will be able to give you your correct BMI and what your ideal weight should be. When you set your overall weight loss goals, this also needs to be realistic. You don't want to get too thin as, once again, you are only going to be playing with your health and well-being.

What Are My Current Commitments?

The above question is more about commitment to your way of life. For example:

- Do you have a family?
    - If you do, you will need to consider what their dietary needs are.
    - How hard will it be to adjust the Atkins eating plan to accommodate them?
    - Don't let this be a stumbling block because it is not that hard to pad carbs for growing children or grown partners. It can even be adjusted to suit the needs of the elderly. Keep in mind that this diet is more about cutting down on carbs and swapping out foods for healthier ones.
- Do you have certain dietary needs?
    - If you have special dietary needs for various reasons, you can work with your health care provider to adjust the Atkins Diet to suit your requirements.
- Do you have any pre-existing conditions?
    - For pre-existing conditions, you should always check with your doctor before starting a new eating plan, no matter what it is.

- o Your doctor will help you or put you in touch with the right person to help you adjust the Atkins Diet to suit your needs.
- Is there anything in your current lifestyle that will stop you from implementing your new lifestyle change?
  - o This could be anything from resistance from your family.
  - o Pressures at work.
  - o Turmoil in your personal life.
  - o Financial issues.
  - o Once you have these listed down try and work in a plan of how you can overcome these obstacles to get you started on the eating plan. Even if you start off making small changes, you will have made a start.

Do I Need Nutritional Supplements?

Every diet needs the recommended daily dosage of vitamins and antioxidants. Even when a person is on a well-balanced diet, they may not be getting enough of these vital nutrients.

Although it is good practice to take multivitamins or certain supplements, always check with a medical professional first. Some medical conditions may be affected by certain substances in supplements.

There are many different multivitamins on the market. The one you choose will depend on your nutrient needs. Some of the essential nutrients the body needs are:

- **Biotin** — Biotin is sometimes referred to as vitamin H or vitamin B7 and it is vital for good skin, nails, and hair health. It also aids the body in converting some nutrients into energy.
- **Boron** — Although not one of the top essential vitamins, boron plays a role in bone health, testosterone levels, estrogen levels, and it helps the body convert certain minerals and vitamins.
- **Calcium** — Calcium is mainly stored in the teeth and bones as it plays a vital role in maintaining and supporting them. This mineral also plays a part in helping the nervous system distribute messages to and from the brain. It is important for maintaining the fluid movement of the muscles.
- **Chromium** — Your body needs small amounts of chromium to help with insulin

sensitivity, protein breakdown, building muscle, and controlling weight.

- **Folate** — Folate is an essential nutrient that aids your body in the production of genetic material, including DNA.
- **Iodine** — Iodine helps the body's metabolism by making thyroid hormones, which are also essential for the development of the brain and bones.
- **Iron** — The lack of iron is a cause of anemia as iron is needed to help oxygenate the blood and produce red blood cells.
- **Magnesium** — Magnesium helps to produce strong healthy bones and DNA, and it helps to keep your blood pressure and blood sugar regulated.
- **Potassium** — Potassium helps the body's muscles and nervous system to function correctly.
- **Selenium** — Selenium has quite a few vital functions in the body, one of which is protecting it from free radicals.
- **Vitamin A** — Vitamin A has a lot to offer the body, including helping the heart, kidneys, and lung function correctly. Beta-carotene is part of the Vitamin A family and it actively helps to keep the immune system healthy, as well as helping with vision.

- **Vitamin B6** — This is a very important vitamin that the body needs to help with various functions such as metabolizing carbohydrates, protein, and fats. It is also needed for the production of neurotransmitters and red blood cells.
- **Vitamin B12** — Vitamin B12 helps the body create DNA for cells and red blood cells, and it keeps the body's nervous system healthy.
- **Vitamin C** — Vitamin C can also be called ascorbic acid. It provides the body with a lot of help with keeping the skin, hair, and nails healthy. It ensures the blood vessels are healthy and aids in the maintenance of good bone health.
- **Vitamin D** — The sun is the most powerful source of vitamin D. But there are many places where there is not a lot of sunlight all year around. A deficiency of vitamin D can lead to a problem called rickets, which is a bone deformity found in children. This vitamin is essential for strong bones and teeth and to help keep the amount of phosphate and calcium in the body regulated.
- **Vitamin E** — Vitamin E is one of the many vitamins that are essential for good skin

health. It also helps the body fight off the damaging effects caused by free radicals.

- **Vitamin K** — Vitamin K helps with bone health and blood clotting.
- **Zinc** — Zinc is found in all the cells in the body. This is an essential nutrient that helps the body fight off intruders such as viruses and bacteria. It also helps in the production of genetic materials including DNA.

Keep a Progress Journal

Keeping a progress journal will help you keep track of your weekly weight loss. You can also keep a quick list of your favorite foods and their net carbs. You can document the foods you love, can tolerate, and cannot stand. It is also a great place to keep your favorite recipes and the ones you make on your own.

It is also a safe place to jot down how you are feeling and your exercise regime.

Getting Started with the Atkins Diet

In a previous section of this chapter, you read about setting yourself realistic and attainable goals. Goals that will not affect your health while still leaving you feeling healthy and energetic. Once your goals are set and you have your motivation, you are ready to choose the correct Atkins Diet plan to suit your individual needs.

To choose the correct Atkins Diet plan/phase for you, you need to ask yourself:

- Do you want to lose weight or maintain your weight and eat healthier?
- If so, do you have over forty pounds to lose? If you do, you will need to start with Phase 1 — The Induction Phase.
- If you have less than 40 pounds to lose, look at starting at Phase 2 — The Ongoing Weight Loss plan, referred to as OWL for short.
- If you want to maintain your weight and want to live the "Atkins Lifestyle," look at starting at Phase 3 — The Pre-Maintenance Phase.
- Phase 4 is the Lifetime Maintenance Phase of the Atkins Diet program.

Read through the diet and make sure you understand it. If you are uncertain about something, Atkins has a very helpful team of people waiting to answer your questions. Reading through the diet will help you become more familiar with the foods you can eat on the different stages and what to avoid, especially in the Inductions Phase, which is the phase that trains your system to burn fat in your body.

Once you have familiarized yourself with the foods, check your pantry, refrigerator, and freezer to see what items you may already have. Make your grocery list and remember to note the carbs in your regular products. When you are at the grocery store, try to find similar low-carb alternatives.

Chapter 3: Working Through Phase 1 — The Induction Phase of the Atkins Diet

You will find the Atkins diet is easy to embrace and follow once you understand it. In this chapter, you are going to learn about each phase of the Atkins Diet. You will also become more familiar with the foods you can eat in each phase.

Phase 1 is the phase that most people who start the Atkins Diet plan start with. This is the phase where you cut down on your carbohydrate intake. Cutting down and controlling the number of carbohydrates you eat each day retrains the way your body burns fuel. Without the excess carbohydrates to store away, your body will start to burn fat.

Phase 1 is also the hardest part of the diet. I will not lie; the first few days I felt a little off my game. I am coffee-holic for one, so cutting down on my favorite beverage did not help my situation at all. I found drinking a lot of water, going for a walk around the garden, or even doing a few stretches helped. You can even try a bit of fresh mint/spearmint soaked in filtered water for a couple of hours or overnight. I found this helped me with any headaches and cravings and it filled me up.

No matter how hard it gets on Phase 1, the trick is not to quit. One of my favorite sayings is "When you are going through hell, keep going" (Winston Churchill). Push through the first week and the second week will not be that bad.

The Induction Phase of the Atkins diet usually lasts two weeks. You can stay on the Induction Phase for much longer should you need to. You can extend the two-week Induction phase if:

- You feel you have not lost enough weight.
- You are not yet 15 pounds from your goal weight.

Starting Phase 1 — Induction

You must stick to the recommended daily carbohydrates you consume. If you work within the following simple guideline for Phase 1, you will get the results you are hoping for.

- In Phase 1, you can eat 20 grams of **net carbohydrates** per day. When you follow the Atkins Diet, you count grams of Net Carbs, which represent the total carbohydrate content of the food minus the fiber content and sugar alcohols (if in the product). Net carbohydrates (Net Carbs) = Total Carbohydrates - Fiber - Sugar

Alcohols (if applicable). When we will count carbohydrates in our meals, we will always count Net Carbs.

- You can eat less but should never go below 18 grams per day. Always check with a dietician, nutritionist, or health care professional first.
- If you feel you need a few more grams of carbs, try not to go over 22 grams per day. If you are eating 22 grams per day, slowly try to reduce the number of carbs to 20 grams after a week.
- Divide your 20 grams of carbohydrates into the following:
  ○ Acceptable salad or cooked vegetable — Eat 12-15 grams per day.
- Limit your protein: ideally consume a moderate amount of protein foods - such poultry, meat, fish or eggs - in each meal and that equates to 115-175g (in weight) or 4-6oz.
- You need to keep yourself hydrated by drinking at least eight glasses of water per day. It is natural for your body to lose water weight on a diet. This can lead a person to feel dizzy, lightheaded, or lacking energy. Keeping yourself hydrated is the key to counteracting this.

- It is important to eat three square meals a day.
- Do not skip meals or snacks. If you are not hungry at mealtime, rather have a small snack or appetizer. Skipping a meal could make you overeat at the next one.
- You can also eat four to five small meals per day if you are used to eating more than three meals a day. Try eating three meals with a snack in between each meal.
- Try not to go without eating for longer than six hours at a time. You should try to eat something every three to four hours.
- Do not overeat. Eat until you feel full and no more. If you have eaten your meal or snack and still feel hungry, have a glass of water.
- Be aware of hidden sugars in some low-carb foods. Always read the nutritional labels.
- In Phase 1, fruit is not recommended; instead, all the nutrients you need are gained from the vegetables and other acceptable foods that are listed below.
- For the first two weeks of the Atkins Diet, seeds and nuts are not on the acceptable foods list and should be avoided.
- Chickpeas, legumes, kidney beans, and similar foods that are a mix of proteins and carbohydrates should be avoided.

- It is advisable to take a multivitamin to ensure you are getting all the nutrients your body needs. This is especially true during this phase of the diet when your body is adjusting to the change in your eating habits.
- You can enjoy fats on the Atkins diet as it is essential for helping the body to absorb various vitamins.
- Try and cut down on how much you eat during meal and snack times. If you still feel hungry after a meal, have a glass of water or a low-carb snack. Keep in mind that the snack will add to your carb intake for the day.
- Try to cut back on the amount of caffeine you drink per day. You need to become aware of what products contain caffeine as well.
- Be careful using or consuming too much artificial sugar substitutes. A lot of them are harmful, can have a laxative effect, and some even contain carbs (up to 1 g per packet).

What You Can Eat

The table below lists the food groups and recommended daily or weekly amounts. The recommendations below are to help you achieve optimum health. They are also designed to get your body to start using fat as its major fuel source.

Food Group	Description	Amount	Per Day/ Week
Beverages	Be aware of hidden sugars in certain beverages.	64 ounces (8 glasses) of liquid	Day
Dairy	No dairy except for certain cheeses, cream, or butter.	3 to 4 ounces	Day
Dressings	Salad dressings can contain quite a lot of carbs and sugars. Read the labels carefully. Limit dressings and opt to make your own low carb ones.	3 grams or lower	As required
Eggs	Eggs are an excellent source of nutrients. Try to eat at least 1 a day. Keep in mind that	2 to 3 eggs	Day

	1 large boiled egg can contain up to 0.6 grams of carbohydrates.		
Fats and Oils	Fats and oils generally have no to very little carbs. However, there is strict guidance on the recommended daily allowance. Always check if fats or oils are safe to cook with. Certain oils should not reach high temperatures.	2 to 4 tablespoons	Day
Fish	Fish is a good source of many nutrients, protein, and good fats. However, your body needs a variety of proteins so it is a good idea to eat a variety of different meats each week.	4 to 6 ounces	2 to 3 times a week
Garnishes	If you want to garnish a salad or dish, try using low to no carb garnishes.	1 large hard boil egg (0.6 g carbs) ½ cup sautéed mushrooms	As required

		(1 g carbs)	
Herbs	Herbs are a great way to add flavor to a dish. When buying herbs, opt for fresh herbs. You can use dried herbs if you do check the label for any added sugar.	Up to 1 tablespoon	As required
Meat	Use only fresh meat and avoid processed meats. This includes meat such as some bacon products, ham, and other processed cold meats. Be aware of any added nitrates that have been added to meat products.	4 to 6 ounces	2 to 3 times a week
Poultry	Poultry is another good source of protein. Although there are no carbs, like fish, you should only eat it a few times a week.	4 to 6 ounces	2 to 3 times a week
Shellfish	Shellfish is one of	Up to 4	2 to 3

	the best sources of essential nutrients such as zinc, iron, magnesium. It is also a source of Omega fatty acids, protein, and other healthy fats. You should keep in mind that some shellfish contain carbs.	ounces	times a week
Spices	Spices add flavor to any dish. Some spices like cayenne pepper can aid in weight loss. Always check for added sugar when choosing a spice brand. You can use salt but limit it and try to use only a pinch at a time.	Up to 1 tablespoon	As required
Sweeteners	Be wary of sweeteners. Some sweeteners are not good for your health. Opt for the more natural sweeteners like Stevia. One packet can also contain up to	3 packets or teaspoons	Day

	1 g of carbs.		
Vegetables	When you measure vegetables, you need to do so when they are raw. For the first two weeks. stick to the acceptable foods list for the foundation vegetables. Never drop below 12 g of these vegetables per serving if possible.	12 to 15 g	Day

Food List for Phase 1

The following is a list of the acceptable foods for each of the above categories. They contain a basic guide to the recommended portion size and total (net) carbs for each. This list is an excellent reference to help you choose your foods per meal and quickly put together a balanced meal.

Food	Amount	Net Carbs
Beverages		
Almond milk — unflavored and unsweetened	1 cup	1 g
Club soda	1 glass	0 g
Coffee — Decaffeinated or caffeinated (carbs measured for black coffee with no added sugar)	1 cup	0 g
Coconut milk — Unflavored and unsweetened	1 cup	2 g
Cream — Light	3.5 ounces	3.7 g
Diet soda (check the label for hidden sugars)	1 glass	0 g
Soy milk — Unflavored and unsweetened	1 cup	4g
Tea — Regular (carbs measured for black tea with no added sugar)	1 cup	0 g

Tea — Herbal (carbs measured for herbal tea with no added sugar)		
Water — Sparkling, still, mineral, tap, or spring	1 glass	0 g
Dairy		
Blue cheese	1 tablespoon	0.2 g
Cheddar cheese	1 ounce	0.4 g
Cream cheese	1 tablespoon	0.4 g
Feta cheese	1 ounce	1.2 g
Goat cheese	1 ounce	0.3 g
Gouda cheese	1 ounce	0.6 g
Mozzarella cheese	1 ounce	0.6 g
Parmesan cheese — Grated	1 tablespoon	0.2 g
Swiss cheese	1 ounce	1.0 g
Dressings		
Balsamic vinegar	1 tablespoon	2.7 g
Blue cheese salad dressing	1 tablespoon	2.3 g

Caesar salad dressing	1 tablespoon	1 g
Greek salad dressing	1 tablespoon	0.5 g
Italian salad dressing — Creamy	1 tablespoon	1.5 g
Lemon juice	1 tablespoon	1 g
Lime juice	1 tablespoon	1.2 g
Ranch salad dressing	1 tablespoon	0.7 g
Red wine vinegar White wine vinegar	1 tablespoon	0 g
Eggs		
Boiled	1 large egg	0.3 g
Devilled	1 large egg	2 g
Fried	1 large egg	0.6 g
Omelets	1 large egg	0.4 g
Poached	1 large egg	0.4 g
Scrambled	1 large egg	2 g
Fats and Oils		

Butter	1 tablespoon	0 g
Mayonnaise (with no added sugar)	1 tablespoon	0 g
Canola oil Coconut oil Grape seed oil Olive oil Safflower oil Sesame oil Soybean oil Sunflower oil Walnut oil	1 tablespoon	0 g

Fish

Cod Flounder Halibut Herring Salmon Sardines Sole Trout Tuna	4 ounces	0 g

Garnishes

Bacon — Crumbled (make sure there is no added sugar)	3 slices	0 g
Cream — Sour	tablespoon	0.6 g
Egg — Hard boiled	1 large egg	0.6 g

Cheese — Grated (different cheeses have different carb counts)	tablespoon	varies
Mushrooms — Sautéed	½ cup	1 g
Herbs		
Basil, Cilantro, Dill, Oregano, Tarragon	1 tablespoon	0 g
Chives	1 tablespoon	0.1 g
Garlic	1 clove	0.9 g
Ginger	1 tablespoon	0.8 g
Parsley	1 tablespoon	0.1 g
Rosemary	1 tablespoon	0.8 g
Sage	1 teaspoon	0.8 g
Meat		
Bacon	4 ounces	1.6 g
Beef	4 ounces	0 g
Ham	4 ounces	4.3 g
Lamb Pork Veal	4 ounces	0 g

Venison		

Poultry

Chicken Cornish hen Duck Goose Turkey Ostrich	4 ounces	0 g

Shellfish

Clams	4 ounces	0.7 g
Crab	4 ounces	0.5 g
Crayfish, Shrimp, Lobster	4 ounces	0 g
Mussels	4 ounces	3.4 g
Oysters	4 ounces	3.1 g
Squid	4 ounces	0.8 g

Spices

Black pepper	1 teaspoon	0.9 g
Cayenne pepper	1 teaspoon	0 g
Salt — A dash/pinch of salt (0.4g) is 155 mg dietary sodium.	1 pinch	0 g
White pepper	1 teaspoon	0.9 g

Sweeteners — Choose a brand that has zero carbs if you can. 1 Packet = 1 tsp		
Saccharine Stevia Sucralose	1 packet	0 to 1 g
Vegetables		
Alfalfa sprouts — Raw	½ cup	0 g
Artichoke — Pickled/marinated	1	1 g
Arugula — Raw	½ cup	0.2 g
Asparagus — Cooked	6 stalks	1.9 g
Avocado — Raw	½	1.3 g
Beet greens — Cooked	½ cup	1.8 g
Bell pepper green — Raw	½ cup	2.2 g
Bell pepper red — Raw	½ cup	3 g
Bell pepper yellow — Raw	½ cup	3 g
Bok choy — Cooked	½ cup	0.4 g
Broccoli — Cooked	½ cup	1.8 g
Broccoli rabe — Cooked	½ cup	1.2 g
Broccolini — Cooked	3	1.9 g
Brussel sprouts — Cooked	½ cup	3.5 g
Button mushroom — Raw	½ cup	0.8 g

Cabbage — Cooked	½ cup	2.7 g
Cauliflower — Cooked	½ cup	1.7 g
Celery — Raw	1 stalk	1 g
Cherry tomato — Raw	10	4.6 g
Chicory greens — Raw	½ cup	0.1 g
Collard greens — Cooked	½ cup	1 g
Cucumber — Raw	½ cup	1.6 g
Dill pickles	1	1 g
Eggplant — Cooked	½ cup	2.3 g
Endive — Raw	½ cup	0.1 g
Escarole — Raw	½ cup	0.1 g
Fennel — Raw	½ cup	1.8 g
Garlic — Minced	2 tablespoons	5.3 g
Green beans — Cooked	½ cup	2.9 g
Kale — Cooked	½ cup	2.4 g
Kohlrabi — Cooked	½ cup	4.6 g
Leeks — Cooked	2 tablespoons	3.4 g
Lettuce — Raw	½ cup	0.5 g

Okra — Cooked	½ cup	1.8 g
Olives black — Raw	5	0.7 g
Olives green — Raw	5	0.1 g
Onion red/white — Raw	2 tablespoons	1.5 g
Portobello mushroom — Cooked	1	2.6 g
Pumpkin — Cooked	½ cup	4.7 g
Radish — Raw	1	0.2 g
Radish (daikon/white) — Raw (grated)	½ cup	1.4 g
Rhubarb — Raw	½ cup	1.8 g
Sauerkraut — Drained	½ cup	1.2 g
Scallion — Raw	½ cup	2.4 g
Shallot — Raw	2 tablespoons	3.4 g
Snow peas — Cooked	½ cup	5.4 g
Spaghetti squash — Cooked	½ cup	4 g
Spinach — Raw	½ cup	0.2 g
Sprouts/mung beans — Raw	½ cup	2.2 g
Swiss chard — Cooked	½ cup	1.8 g

Tomato small — Raw	1	2.5 g
Turnip greens — Cooked	½ cup	0.6 g
Turnip — Cooked	½ cup	2.4 g
Watercress — Raw	½ cup	0.1 g
Yellow squash — Cooked	½ cup	2.6 g
Zucchini — Cooked	½ cup	1.5 g

What Foods You Should Avoid

When you start with the Induction Phase of the Atkins Diet, there are foods you need to stay away from. The list below will give you a basic outline of which foods are not on the acceptable food and beverage list for Phase 1.

Foods to Avoid for Phase 1

Alcohol
During the Induction Phase, **no alcohol** is allowed. The consumption of alcohol may slow down your weight loss. In Phase 2, you can start to re-introduce a limited amount to your diet plan.
Baked Goods and Desserts
Stay away from all baked goods such as cakes, cookies, biscuits, muffins, pretzels, savory pies, bread, and rolls.

Avoid all kinds of desserts such as puddings, mousse, flan, pies, donuts, and so on.

Dairy
Flavored milk
Ice cream
Milk
Milkshakes
Yogurt drinks
Yogurt — Sweetened/flavored
Diet/Low-Fat Foods
You have to be very careful with foods marked both diet or low-fat.
Low-fat foods may still contain quite a bit of sugar.
Diet foods may still contain a high carb content.
Fruit
No fruit may be eaten during Phase 1.
Grains
Barely
Rice
Rye
Spelt

Wheat

Processed Foods

Processed food has gone through a process such as being ground, cured, rolled, etc.

Potato chips are an example of processed food, chopped ham, most bought baked goods, and so on.

Although some processed foods are not bad for you, you cannot eat them during Phase 1 of the Atkins Diet.

Some examples of **healthier processed** foods are:

Crackers made with whole-grains

Dried fruit

Ground corn tortillas

Frozen vegetables

Pasta made with whole-grains

Pitas made with whole-grains

Pizza bases made with whole-grains

Rice — brown

Rolled oats

Steel-cut oats

Refined Foods

Whole food is a food you can take straight from the garden and eat it. Whole food has a significantly higher nutrient value than its refined counterpart.

Refined food is a food that has been picked/harvested and refined into another form. It will no longer contain the same nutrient value as did in its whole form.

Some examples of refined foods are:

Cakes

Cookies

Pasta — There are some pasta brands that are refined, especially white pasta.

Pastries

Potato chips

Pretzels

Rice — Some rice is refined, especially white rice.

Wheat bread

White flour

White sugar

Wraps

Starchy/High Carb Vegetables/Legumes

You cannot eat starchy vegetables during Phase 1 of the Atkins diet; some examples are starchy vegetables are:

Beans — Black, cannellini, kidney, navy, and pinto

Butternut squash

Carrots
Chickpeas
Corn
Lentils
Parsnips
Peas
Potatoes
Sweet potatoes
Turnips
Yams
Sweetened Beverages
Cordials
Ice coffees/teas
Fizzy flavored sodas
Slushies
Smoothies — high carb
Sweets
All sweets, including shaved ice, ice pops, lollipops, boiled sweets, toffies, chocolates, gummy sweets, mints, chewing gum, etc. should be avoided. If you have a sweet tooth, try a low-carb smoothie, health bar, or low-carb snack.

Meal Plan

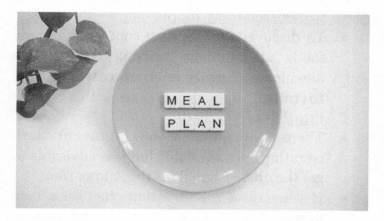

Below is a seven-day example meal plan for Phase 1 of the Atkins Diet. When planning your meals:

- Do not exceed your daily net carb allowance.
- Counting your net carbs:
  - Net carbs = Total Carbohydrates - Fiber
  - If there is Sugar Alcohols listed, the calculation will be:
    - Net carbs = Total Carbohydrates - Fiber - Sugar Alcohols
- You can calculate your net carbs by using the "Net Carb Calculator," which you can download onto an Android or iOS mobile device. You can find the app in your mobile

application store or go to the Atkins website: https://www.atkins.com/how-it-works/free-tools/mobile-app

- To discover the net carb count of as many foods as humanly possible - You can download a **handy carb counter in PDF format** by going to this link: http://bit.ly/carbpdf
- There are quite a few different carb counting apps available but it is advisable to get the one designed for the Atkins Diet.
- If you are at a loss, Atkins has their own brand of foods that are quick and easy to make. They offer Atkins Frozen Food and Meals, Atkins Bar, Atkins Shake, Atkins Treats, and more.
- The Atkins website provides useful information about where to buy their diet products from: https://www.atkins.com/products.
- Some large chain stores and Amazon also stock certain Atkins products. Always make sure you are buying true Atkins products when purchasing from the internet.

Phase 1 Seven-Day Meal Plan Example

Drink at least eight glasses of water a day to keep yourself hydrated.

Monday	
Breakfast	2 eggs, scrambled Served with: 2 oz smoked salmon ¼ tsp black pepper 1/2 avocado
Snack	1 Pepperoni stick
Lunch	A mixed green salad consisting of: 5 green olives 1.3 oz feta cheese 3 cherry tomatoes ½ tbsp white wine vinegar and 1 tbsp virgin olive oil dressing Topped with: 3 slices of crumbled bacon garnish
Snack	1 celery stalk stuffed with 2 tbsp of cream cheese
Dinner	3 oz tuna Mixed with: 1 tbsp mayonnaise 2 tbsp baby spinach, chopped 1 tbsp cheddar cheese — grated Baked for 8 to 10 minutes on: 2 portobello mushrooms
Tuesday	
Breakfast	2-egg omelet Filled with: 2 tbsp grated cheddar cheese 2 tbsp chopped spinach leaves 3 cherry tomatoes

Snack	Atkins snack bar — Peanut Butter Protein Wafer Crisps
Lunch	2 oz ground beef burger patty Cooked with: 1 oz grated cheddar cheese 1 tbsp white onions finely chopped Served on: ½ cup cauliflower — grated
Snack	1 grilled chicken leg
Dinner	2 poached eggs Served in: 1 Hass avocado (medium) — halved Topped with: 2 oz smoked salmon 1 tsp dill ¼ tsp black pepper
Wednesday	
Breakfast	2 boiled eggs Served with: 3 slices of cooked bacon 4 cherry tomatoes Fried in: 2 tsp vegetable or coconut oil
Snack	1 oz string cheese
Lunch	2 oz lean beef strips Stir-fried with: 1 tbsp shallots — chopped ½ cup broccoli ½ cup eggplant — cubed
Snack	4 cherry tomatoes

	Topped with: 1 tbsp grated mozzarella ¼ tsp fresh basil dash of black pepper Grill for 5 to 8 minutes
Dinner	3 oz lean chicken breast Grilled with: ¼ tsp fresh crushed garlic ¼ cup of button mushrooms a dash of black pepper Served with: ½ cup cooked spaghetti squash
Thursday	
Breakfast	3 oz smoked salmon Served with: ¼ cup cucumber — chopped 1 tbsp cream cheese
Snack	½ avocado, Hass
Lunch	2 oz shrimp Served with: ¼ cup crisp lettuce leaves — shredded 2 green olives 2 black olives 1 tbsp cucumber — julienned 2 tsp mayonnaise
Snack	1 medium red bell pepper Stuffed with: 1 tbsp cream cheese Topped with: ¼ tsp dill a dash of black pepper

Dinner	2 oz trout Grilled with: 3 cherry tomatoes ¼ tsp crushed garlic dash of black pepper Served with: green leaf salad drizzle with a dressing made up of: 3 tsp olive oil 1 tsp white wine vinegar 1 tsp fresh chopped basil 1 packet of Stevia
Friday	
Breakfast	2 egg omelet Stuffed with: 1 tbsp vegetables of your choice from the approved vegetable list 1 tbsp grated cheddar cheese
Snack	Atkins Vanilla Latte Iced Coffee Protein Shake
Lunch	meatballs Served on: ½ cup mashed cauliflower
Snack	1 oz string cheese
Dinner	Pork chops — grilled ½ cup mixed vegetables from the approved vegetable list
Saturday	
Breakfast	½ avocado, Hass

	Topped with: 1 tbsp cream cheese dash of black pepper ½ tsp fresh basil — chopped 3 slices of lean bacon — diced
Snack	1 celery stalk Stuffed with: 1 tbsp cream cheese
Lunch	2 oz lean beef strips Sautéed with: a dash of black pepper ½ portobello mushroom — chopped 1 tbsp green bell pepper — chopped
Snack	Atkins snack bar - the low-carb pick of your choice
Dinner	Chicken salad, mix together: ¼ cup lettuce — shredded 4 green olives 1 tbsp feta cheese 1 tsp watercress 1 tbsp arugula (rocket) ¼ avocado — cubed 2 oz grilled white chicken meat — shredded Drizzle with: 1 tbsp olive oil 2 tsp red wine vinegar dash of cayenne pepper 1 tsp fresh crushed basil
Sunday	
Breakfast	2 boiled eggs Mashed with:

	2 tbsp grilled/microwaved button mushrooms 3 cherry tomatoes A dash of black pepper
Snack	1 Pepperoni stick
Lunch	2 oz roast chicken ½ cup mixed vegetables from the approved vegetable list
Snack	Atkins Chocolate Banana Shake
Dinner	Leftover roast chicken kebabs ½ cup of mixed vegetables from the approved vegetable list

Adding to the Diet's Benefits with Exercises for Phase 1

The Atkins Diet is effective without exercise; however, it is encouraged, and if you can exercise, it can be beneficial to both weight loss and your health. There are many benefits to adding an exercise routine to your day, especially when you are on a diet.

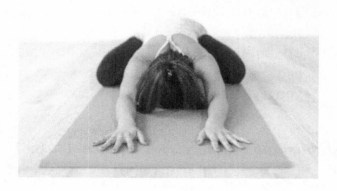

Benefits of Exercise

The benefits of exercising are many-fold. Exercise helps:

- Your body burns fats.
- You achieve your weight loss goal.
- You maintain your optimal weight goal.

- You build muscle to tone your body.
- Maintain healthy joints, bones, and muscle tissue.
- Reduce the risk of developing diseases such as heart disease, diabetes, and high blood pressure.
- Reduce the risk of high cholesterol as it helps to maintain cholesterol levels in the body.
- With depression and anxiety.
- Control a person's stress levels.
- To have a positive effect on a person's psychological well-being.
- To improve a person's self-confidence. It can cut down on mood swings and make you feel more energetic and alert.

Establishing an Exercise Routine in Phase 1

If you have not exercised before or have not exercised for a while, you will need to ease into exercising. If you have any pre-existing conditions, you should check with your doctor first and consult with a trained physical fitness instructor. There are many benefits to exercising but, at the same time, you need to know your body's limitations.

Although focusing on getting your body into peak physical condition is something to work towards, you do not have to kill yourself to get there. For someone who is into sports or competes at a high level, their bodies are trained to be exercising machines. Most normal people may go for a hike, or take a walk, play a bit of tennis, or go for a jog. You are not looking to win any competitions or become a sports star.

There has been a lot of research over the last few decades that have shown even light exercise has benefits (Metcalfe, 2019). You don't have to become a cardio ninja to increase your body into a fitter state. If you want to become a fitness goddess, then you will need to focus on intense cardio workout mixed with weights, etc.

But, to start with, you can try a few of these exercises to build up your strength:

- To start, you should set your goal for 15 to 20 minutes a day, at least two to three times a week.
- Gradually increase this to 30 minutes a day and a few more days a week.
- Always do at least three to five minutes of stretching before you begin any type of exercise.

- Take a brisk 15 to 20-minute walk once or twice a day. Walking the dogs is good exercise.
- Taking a hike that has dips and inclines for 10 to 20 minutes. Be careful of the terrain you choose and always make sure you have someone with you.
- Do some gardening for 30 minutes; even raking, weeding, and digging are physical activities that can increase your fitness level.
- Do laps in a pool for 10 to 20 minutes as swimming is fun and excellent exercise.
- Cycling for 10 to 15 minutes is excellent for getting your heart rate to increase and working those muscles.
- Yoga or pilates is light, can be relaxing, and is an excellent way to relieve stress, anxiety, as it relaxes you.

Find a workout or type of exercise you enjoy. It does not have to be high impact as long as it gets you moving and your blood flowing. As mentioned above, a stroll around the garden twice a day to water your plants or do some planting also counts as exercise, as does raking the garden.

Playing and being active with the kids is another way to get some exercise in. Then there are exercises you can do while sitting down. These are low-impact callanetic type exercises. If you have stairs in your house, you take a walk up and down them a few times. Instead of taking your car to the market cycle or walk there, as long as it is safe to do so, that is. Every little helps and the more active you get, the more active you will want to become.

Chapter 4: Working Through Phase 2 — Continued Weight Loss Phase of the Atkins Diet

Phase 2 is the phase that builds your daily allowed carb count up a bit. You can start to introduce some foods and beverages that you could not eat in Phase 1 into your daily diet.

The Continued Weight Loss Phase of the Atkins diet usually lasts one to two weeks. Phase 2 should last up until you are within 10 pounds of your goal weight.

Progressing to Phase 2 — Continued Weight Loss

As in Phase 1 of the Atkins Diet plan, in Phase 2, it is important that you stick to the recommended daily carbohydrate goal. Below are a few simple guidelines to help make the transition from Phase 1 to Phase 2 as simple as possible:

- In Phase 2, you can eat 25 grams of carbohydrates per day.
- You can eat less but should never go below 18 grams per day.

- Remember to check with a dietician, nutritionist, or health care professional first before starting any new diet regime. If you have any pre-existing conditions, even transitioning from one phase of the diet to the next should be carefully monitored.
- Try not to exceed your daily carb limit as your body should be used to 20 grams a day by this phase of the diet. If you feel hungry, try drinking a glass of water or eating a no/low-carb snack.
- Divide your 20 grams of carbohydrates into the following:
  - Acceptable salad or cooked vegetable — Eat 12-15 grams per day.
- Limit your protein: ideally consume a moderate amount of protein foods - such poultry, meat, fish or eggs - in each meal and that equates to 115-175g (in weight) or 4-6oz.
- Hydration is still key to keeping yourself from feeling hunger, dizzy, lightheaded, and maintaining good health.
- You still need to eat either three meals a day or four to five smaller ones.
- Have at least one to two low-carb or zero-carb snacks a day in between meals.

- Do not skip your meals even if you only have a snack at mealtime should you not feel hungry.
- Try to eat every three to four hours, once again even if it is just a light snack or low-carb to a zero-carb smoothie.
- Do not overeat during any meal or snack time; remember water fills you up nicely.
- In Phase 2, you can start to introduce various fruits back into your diet plan.
- In Phase 2, you can start to introduce a limited number of nuts and seeds back into your diet plan.
- In Phase 2, you can start to introduce moderate alcoholic drinks back into your diet plan.
- Keeping control of your portion size is highly recommended and will keep the pounds from coming back.
- The Atkins Diet does not recommend caffeine but still allows it in moderation.
- Try not to use a lot of salt, salt products, and artificial sweeteners.

What You Can Eat

The table below lists the food groups and recommended daily or weekly amounts for Phase 2 of the Atkins Diet. The food groups listed below are in addition to the food groups listed in Phase 1.

Food Group	Description	Amount	Per Day/ Week
Alcohol	Limit alcohol. Use diet/carb-free drink mixes. Drink a glass of water before drinking alcohol as it can dehydrate you. Opt for spirits, red or white wines.	1 small glass	Day
Beverages	Always opt for water as your beverage of choice.	64 ounces (8 glasses) of liquid	Day
Dairy	You can add a few more dairy items to the list of approved food for Phase 2.	Varies depending on the type of dairy	Day
Dressings	Salad dressings — same as in Phase 1	3 grams or lower	As required
Eggs	Eggs — same as in Phase 1	2 to 3 eggs	Day
Fats and Oils	Fats and oils — same as in Phase 1	2 to 4 tablespoons	Day
Fish	Fish — same as in Phase 1	4 to 6 ounces	2 to 3 times a

			week
Fruit	You can introduce certain fruits to your diet in Phase 2.	¼ cup	Day/we ek
Garnishes	Garnishes — same as in Phase 1	1 large hard boiled egg (0.6 g carbs) ½ cup sautéed mushrooms (1 g carbs)	As require d
Herbs	Herbs — same as in Phase 1	Up to 1 tablespoon	As require d
Juices	There are certain fruit juices that you can start adding to your diet in Phase 2.	2 tablespoons	As require d
Legumes	Legumes can be added to your diet. These can be cooked or canned.	Varies depending on the type of legume	Day/we ek
Meat	Meat — same as in Phase 1	4 to 6 ounces	2 to 3 times a week
Nuts	Various nuts are allowed in Phase 2 of the diet.	Varies depending on the type of nut	Week
Poultry	Poultry — same as in	4 to 6	2 to 3

	Phase 1	ounces	times a week
Seeds	There are certain seeds you can eat in Phase 2 of the diet.	Varies depending on the type of seed	Week
Shellfish	Shellfish — same as in Phase 1	Up to 4 ounces	2 to 3 times a week
Spices	Spices — same as in Phase 1	Up to 1 tablespoon	As require d
Sweetener s	Sweeteners — same as in Phase 1	3 packets or teaspoons	Day
Vegetables	Vegetables — same as in Phase 1 Legumes can be eaten; please refer to Legumes below.	12 to 15 grams	Day

Food List for Phase 2

The following is a list of the acceptable foods for each of the above categories that you can enjoy in Phase 2 of the Atkins Diet. Please note that these foods are in addition to the food list laid out in Phase 1.

Food	Amount	Net Carbs
Alcohol		
Brandy Bourbon Gin Rum Scotch Whisky Vodka	1.5 fl. oz	0 g
Sherry — Dry	1.5 fl. oz	2 g
Red wine	6 fl. oz	2 g
White wine	6 fl. oz	1 g
Beverages		
All beverages in Phase 1 apply to Phase 2.		
Use diet beverages as mixes for alcohol	1 glass	0 g
Use diet tonic as a mix for alcohol	1 glass	varies
Dairy		
All dairy in Phase 1 apply to Phase 2.		

Cottage cheese (2%)	½ cup	4.1 g
Heavy cream	¾ cup	4.8 g
Ricotta cheese	½ cup	3.8 g
Yogurt — unsweetened, whole milk, Greek	½ cup	3.5 g
Yogurt — unsweetened, whole milk, plain	½ cup	5.5 g

Dressings, Eggs, Fats and Oils, and Fish

All the above food groups listed in Phase 1 apply to Phase 2.

Fruit

Blackberries	¼ cup	1.6 g
Blueberries	¼ cup	4.5 g
Boysenberries	¼ cup	4.5 g
Cantaloupe	¼ cup	2.9 g
Coconut — unsweetened shredded/fresh	¼ cup	2.3 g
Cranberries	¼ cup	1.9 g

Gooseberries	¼ cup	3.9 g
Honeydew	¼ cup	3.5 g
Raspberries	¼ cup	1.7 g

Garnishes, Herbs, Meat, Poultry, Shellfish, Spices, Sweeteners, and Vegetables

All the above food groups listed in Phase 1 apply to Phase 2.

Juices

Lemon juice	2 tablespoons	2 g
Lime juice	2 tablespoons	2.4 g
Tomato juice	4 ounces	4 g

Legumes

Black beans	¼ cup	6.5 g
Chickpeas	¼ cup	10.9 g
Great northern beans	¼ cup	10.6 g
Kidney beans	¼ cup	5.9 g
Lima beans	¼ cup	6.1 g
Navy beans	¼ cup	10.1

Pinto beans	¼ cup	6.1 g

Nuts

Almonds	24 nuts	2.2 g
Brazil nuts	6 nuts	1.4 g
Cashews	2 tablespoons	5.1 g
Macadamias	10 nuts	1.4 g
Peanuts	2 tablespoons	3.8 g
Pecans	2 tablespoons	3.8 g
Pine nuts	2 tablespoons	2 g
Pistachios	2 tablespoons	3 g
Walnuts	12 nuts	1.7 g

Seeds

Pumpkin seeds	2 tablespoons	2 g
Sesame seeds	2 tablespoons	2 g
Sunflower seeds — hulled	2 tablespoons	1.5 g

What Foods You Should Avoid

In Phase 2, there are a few foods that you can start to introduce into your diet plan. However, there are still many foods you need to avoid; the table below lists the foods that you should avoid.

Foods to Avoid for Phase 2

Alcohol
As you read in the acceptable foods list above, during this phase you can start to enjoy certain alcoholic beverages in moderations. You should, however, avoid the following alcoholic beverages:
Alcoholic coffees
Alcoholic iced coffees
Alcoholic ice-creams
Alcoholic milkshakes
Ale — Both dark and light ale
Beer — Including light beers/ non-alcoholic beer
Brandy
Champagne
Cider
Cocktails
Cream-based liqueurs

Dessert wines
Liqueurs
Mocktails
Port
Sherry
Sparkling wines
Stout
Baked Goods and Desserts
You will still need to stay away from the baked goods listed in Phase 1.
With a higher carb intake, you can make low-carb desserts that fit within your daily carb allowance.
Dairy
You will still need to stay away from the dairy items listed in foods to avoid in Phase 1.
Diet/Low-Fat Foods
Always check for hidden sugars in any low-fat or diet food.
Fruit
Only eat the fruits on the approved food list for Phase 2.
Grains
You need to stay away from the grains as listed in foods to avoid in Phase 1.

Processed Foods
You need to stay away from all processed foods as listed in foods to avoid in Phase 1.
Refined Foods
You need to stay away from refined foods as listed in foods to avoid in Phase 1.
Starchy/High Carb Vegetables/Legumes
Only eat the higher carb vegetables and legumes that are listed in the approved food list for phase 2.
Sweetened Beverages
You must avoid any sweetened beverages as listed in Phase 1 foods to avoid list.
Sweets
You still cannot eat any sweets and the same rules apply as listed in the sweets to avoid in Phase 1.
For a sweet tooth, try one of the Atkins low-carb snack bars.

Meal Plan

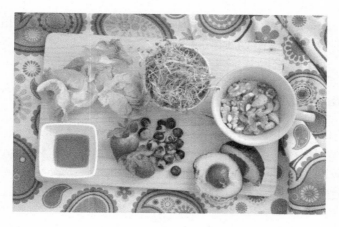

Below is a seven-day example meal plan for Phase 2 of the Atkins Diet. When planning your meals:

- Do not exceed your daily net carb allowance of 25 g per day.
- Try to vary your protein sources each day and week.
- Counting your net carbs:
  - Net carbs = Total Carbohydrates - Fiber
  - If there is Sugar Alcohols listed, the calculation will be:
    - Net carbs = Total Carbohydrates - Fiber - Sugar Alcohols
- You can download various apps from your mobile device's app store.
- You can download the Atkins Net Carb Calculator app from the Atkins website. (All

the information is listed in the Meal Plan section of Phase 1.)

Phase 2 Seven-Day Meal Plan Example

Drink at least eight glasses of water a day. It is important for your optimum health to stay hydrated.

	Monday
Breakfast	Pumpkin, Almond, and Vanilla Whey Protein Sour Cream Pancakes (see Recipe 7)
Snack	6 Brazil nuts and 12 walnuts
Lunch	2 oz ground beef burger patty Topped with: ½ Hass avocado — sliced 1 slice tomato 1 slice cheddar cheese 2 tsp mayonnaise Serve between: 2 grilled portobello mushrooms
Snack	Atkins low-carb shake (no more than 4 g carbs)
Dinner	1.5 oz lamb steak — grilled Served with: 3 oz of cauliflower — mashed Mashed with: 2 tbsp cheddar cheese — grated 2 slices of fresh tomato A dash of ground black pepper 1 tsp mustard

Tuesday	
Breakfast	2 Atkins crisp bread Topped with: ½ Hass avocado — sliced 4 slices of cucumber 1 tbsp feta cheese — crumbled a dash of black pepper drizzled with lemon juice
Snack	2 oz Greek yogurt 1 tbsp blueberries
Lunch	2 oz salmon fillet — grilled 2 tbsp feta cheese — crumbled 1 tbsp cashew nuts Served on: ¼ baby spinach leaves a dash of ground black pepper
Snack	¼ honeydew melon
Dinner	2 oz roasted chicken Served with: ¼ cup pumpkin — cooked ¼ cup Brussels sprouts — cooked 1 portobello mushroom — grilled ¼ tsp crushed garlic a dash of cayenne pepper
Wednesday	
Breakfast	Chocolate, Mint, and Avocado Smoothie (see Recipe 32)

Snack	Atkins snack (no more than 4 g net carbs)
Lunch	Salad made with: ¼ baby spinach leaves 2 tbsp feta cheese 1 tbsp raspberries 1 tbsp blueberries 1 tsp pine nuts Salad dressing made from: 1 tbsp white wine vinegar 1 tsp olive oil 1 tsp fresh basil 2 packets of Stevia
Snack	¼ cup strawberries
Dinner	Vegetable Lamb Stew (see Recipe 19)
Thursday	
Breakfast	2-egg omelet Filled with: 1 oz smoked salmon ½ tsp capers 1 tsp dill ¼ tsp cayenne pepper 2 tbsp feta cheese — crumbled
Snack	¼ cup strawberries
Lunch	2 oz grilled chicken — shredded Mixed into the following salad: ¼ cup brown mushrooms — sautéed ¼ cup baby spinach leaves — shredded ¼ cup iceberg lettuce leaves — shredded 2 tbsp blue cheese — crumbled (replace with feta if desired) 1 tsp roasted sesame seeds

	Topped with the following dressing: 1 tsp olive oil 3 tsp red wine vinegar a dash of ground black pepper
Snack	Atkins Iced Coffee Milkshake
Dinner	Chicken kebabs made from: 3 oz grilled white chicken meat — cubed ¼ cup red bell pepper — sliced ¼ cup shallots — sliced ¼ cup brown mushrooms — halved Place chicken and vegetables onto kebab sticks and grill. Serve on a bed of: ¼ cup baby spinach — slightly cooked
Friday	
Breakfast	2 eggs — scrambled Scrambled with: 1 tbsp scallions — chopped 1 tbsp fresh baby spinach — shredded 1 tbsp cheddar cheese — shredded 1 tbsp feta cheese — crumbled
Snack	1 Atkins crisp bread Topped with: 1 tbsp chunky cottage cheese 3 green pitted olives — halved a dash of cayenne pepper
Lunch	Artichoke and Sesame Seed Salad (see Recipe 9)
Snack	12 walnuts and 1 tsp sesame seeds
Dinner	Beef Stroganoff on a Bed of Green Bean (see

	Recipe 15)
Saturday	
Breakfast	Berry Coconut Breakfast Parfait (see Recipe 5)
Snack	1 tbsp honeydew melon and 1 tbsp cranberries or raspberries
Lunch	Hearty Cream of Asparagus Soup (see Recipe 12)
Snack	Atkins snack (no more than 4 g net carbs)
Dinner	Filet Medallions with Blackberry, Feta, and Spinach Salad (see Recipe 16)
Sunday	
Breakfast	Breakfast Blueberry Muffins (see Recipe 3)
Snack	Atkins shake — a flavor of your choice (no more than 4 g net carbs)
Lunch	Portobello Beef Burger with Feta and Spring Onion (see Recipe 14)
Snack	1 tbsp pumpkin seeds
Dinner	Lamb Chops with Cauliflower Mash (see Recipe 17)

Adding to the Diet's Benefits with Exercises for Phase 2

If you have been exercising through Phase 1, you should, by now, be ready to slightly increase your routine. That is if you are physically able to and there are not any issues that prevent you from doing so.

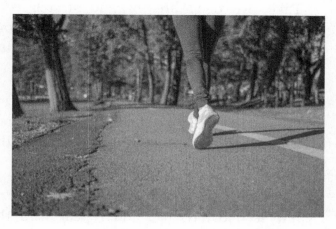

You may want to try to include the following few exercises into your routine:

- **Stretch**

    Start with a three to five-minute stretch. You can either lie on the floor on a mat. Lift your arms over your head and stretch your legs out. Point your toes to feel the stretch in your calves.

Bring your arms down and lift one knee to your chest. Hold for five seconds and repeat the stretch with your other knee.

Roll up into a sitting position with your legs folded in front of you. Roll your neck to one side, then pivot it around the back to the other side and roll it around the front.

Take two deep breaths and stretch your arms up above your head, then out in front of you, before rolling into a standing position.

Take a deep breath and stretch your arms up as if you can lift yourself up on your toes as you stretch. Breathe out and relax the stretch; repeat one more time.

Lift your foot up to your buttocks, hold for a few seconds, release and repeat with the other leg. If you cannot balance, make sure to hold onto a firm structure for support.

Remember to stretch after you have exercised as well.

- **Arm rolls**

  To firm up your arms, hold your arms out to the sides with your fingers up. Rotate your arms around in small circles 20 times backward and 20 times forward. You can gradually increase these as you feel you can do more.

- **Squats**

  Hold on to the back of a chair if you are unable to balance. Make sure your feet are planted firmly on the floor and facing forward but slightly apart. Keep your back straight, head up, then squat. Sink into the squat like you are about to sit on a chair. Do 5 to 10 repetitions and gradually increase these as your strength improves.

- **Crunches**

  Standing crunches are just as good as the ones you do lying down. Stand with your buttocks squeezed tight and shoulders back. Suck your tummy in. Put your arms out in front of you. As you pull your arms back towards your body, ball your hands into fists as if you are pulling a weight. Tilt your pelvis forward, make sure to suck in your tummy. You should feel the stretch in your belly. Hold for two seconds, release, and repeat for 20 to 30 crunches.

For lying down crunches, position a mat on the floor. Lie down flat on the mat. Pull your knees up and suck your belly in picturing your belly button pulling towards your spine. Place your hands behind your head and tilt your chin towards your chest.

Do NOT pull your crunch up with your arms as this only strains your neck. You need to feel the crunch by using your stomach muscles to lift your upper body. Do not swing into a full sit-up either. You need to gently lift your upper body until your shoulders are not on the floor. Keep your buttocks tight, tummy sucked in, and your lower back on the floor. Hold the crunch of a second before releasing it.

Do 5 to 10 of these and gradually increase the number of crunches as you feel stronger. Remember, if you can feel the crunch in your neck, you are pulling up wrong. Your head and neck should remain relaxed while you are crunching.

- **Push-Ups**

You are probably thinking *"Agh, I hate those"*; well these are push-ups with a difference. To increase your arm strength, you can lean against a sturdy counter or even a wall. It is best to start off with the wall.

Stand with your palms flat against the wall and an arm's length away from the wall. Your feet should be shoulder-width apart and facing forward. Keep your shoulders straight, chin up, and buttocks and stomach must be pulled tight. Allowing your full weight to lean in towards the wall. It is like doing a push-up standing up. Make sure to bend your elbows as you lean forward, pull them in against your body.

Push away from the wall, straightening your elbows as you stand back up straight. Do not remove your hands from the wall. Repeat the process for 10 to 15 repetitions, which you can increase as your strength does.

For a harder version of this push-up: lean at a slight angle against a countertop. But make sure your feet are flat on the floor.

Well done! You have worked hard to get through the second phase of the Atkins diet. Keep going you are closing in on your goals.

Chapter 5: Phase 3 — Pre-Maintenance Phase of the Atkins Diet

If you have advanced to Phase 3, congratulations as you should only have approximately 10 pounds to lose to reach your goal weight. You can also go straight to phase 3 without phases 1 and 2 if you only have 10 pounds or less to lose.

Continuing on to Phase 3 — Pre-Maintenance

Phase 3 is called the Pre-Maintenance Phase as it is designed to get you to your goal weight, and then help you maintain that weight for at least four weeks. This means that this phase can last from six to eight weeks, depending on how rapidly you drop those last few extra pounds.

- In Phase 3, you can eat 30 grams of carbohydrates per day until you have lost your desired weight.
- Once you have reached your goal weight, you need to maintain that weight for at least four weeks thereafter.

- During those four weeks, you need to slightly increase your carbohydrate intake by 5 to 10 grams a day each week.
- By the time you are ready to progress to Phase 4, you should be eating approximately 80 to 100 grams of carbohydrates a day. This amount depends on how your body responds to the higher carb rate. If you feel you are putting on weight, drop the amount down by 5 grams.
- As you introduce more starchy foods into your body, you will be able to figure out how your body responds to them. If you feel bloated or uncomfortable, you know to leave that food out altogether. Watch your carb count closely when introducing higher carb foods.
- Before you start a new phase of the Atkins Diet, always check with a dietician, nutritionist, or health care professional. This will ensure you can apply to continue with the plan or if you need to adjust the diet.
- Try not to go over your set daily allowed carbohydrate consumption.
- Your daily amount of carbohydrates should include 12 to 15 grams of acceptable foods and vegetables.

- Limit your protein: ideally consume a moderate amount of protein foods - such poultry, meat, fish or eggs - in each meal and that equates to 115-175g (in weight) or 4-6oz.
- Drink at least eight glasses of water per day.
- Eating three square meals a day is a must and you should not skip meals or snacks.
- Eat four to five smaller meals a day rather than three if you find this helps stave off hunger and stops any cravings.
- Try and eat something every three to four hours. Never go longer than six hours without eating.
- Always be on the lookout for hidden sugars in all foods and beverages.
- Keep your portion size down to the amount that leaves you feeling full. You don't want to feel like you are stuffed or bloated after a meal.
- Don't overeat; eat until you're full.
- Keep alcohol and caffeine to a minimum.

What You Can Eat

The food groups for Phase 3 remain the same as they were in Phase 2. However, there are a few foods that can be reintroduced into your diet plan in this Phase.

Acceptable Food List for Phase 3

The following is a list of the acceptable foods that you can enjoy in Phase 3 of the Atkins Diet. Please note that these foods are in addition to the food lists laid out in Phase 1 and Phase 2.

Food	Amount	Net Carbs
Alcohol		
All acceptable alcohol in Phase 2 applies to Phase 3.		
Beverages, Dairy, Dressings, Eggs, Fats and Oils, Fish, Garnishes, Herbs, Juices, Legumes, Meat, Poultry, Shellfish, Spices, Sweeteners, and Vegetables.		
All the above food groups listed in Phase 1 and Phase 2 apply to Phase 3.		
Fruit		
All fruit in Phase 1 and 2 apply to Phase 3.		
Apple	½ fruit	7.9 g
Apricot — medium	3 fruit	9.6 g

Banana — small	1 fruit	20.4 g
Cherries	¼ cup	5.3 g
Clementine	1 fruit	7.6 g
Coconut — fresh and unsweetened shredded	½ cup	2.5 g
Dates — fresh	3 fruit	15.8 g
Figs — fresh	1 fruit	4.5 g
Grapes — red	½ cup	13 g
Grapefruit — medium	½ fruit	8.9 g
Guava	½ cup	7.4 g
Kiwi	1 fruit	8.1 g
Mango	½ cup	11.1 g
Orange	½ cup	14.5 g
Papaya	½ cup	6.6 g

Peach — small	1 fruit	10.5 g
Pineapple	½ cup	9.7 g
Plum — medium	1 fruit	6.6 g
Pomegranate seeds	¼ cup	6.4 g
Watermelon	½ cup	5.5 g
Grains — amounts can vary depending on the brand		
Barley — cooked	½ cup	19.2 g
Bread — whole wheat	2 slices	20 g
Grits — cooked	½ cup	15.2 g
Millet — cooked	½ cup	19.5 g
Oat bran	2 tablespoons	6.0 g
Oatmeal	⅓ cup	19 g
Pasta — whole wheat and cooked	½ cup	16.6 g

Polenta	2 tablespoons	12.5 g
Quinoa — cooked	¼ cup	8.6 g
Rice — brown and cooked	½ cup	21.2 g
Wheat bran	2 tablespoons	1.6 g
Wheat germ	2 tablespoons	4.9 g

Nuts

All nuts in Phase 1 and 2 apply to Phase 3.

Pine Nuts	2 tablespoons	0.8 g

Poultry

All poultry in Phase 1 and 2 apply to Phase 3.

Seeds

All seeds in Phase 1 and 2 apply to Phase 3.

Poppy seeds	1 tablespoon	1.2 g
Pumpkin seeds	2 tablespoons	2.4 g

Sesame seeds	2 tablespoons	2.1 g

Vegetables — Starchy

Acorn squash	½ cup	7.6 g
Beets	½ cup	6.8 g
Butternut squash	½ cup	8.5 g
Carrots	½ cup	4 g
Corn	½ cup	14.9 g
Parsnips	½ cup	10.2 g
Peas	½ cup	7 g
Potato — baked, medium	½ potato	13.1 g
Sweet potato — baked, medium	½ potato	9.9 g
Rutabaga	½ cup	5.9 g

What Foods You Should Avoid

Phase 3 is a little more lenient with the foods you may eat as long as you watch your crabs and remain within your daily allowance. You should still stay away from the obvious foods such as sugary sweets, drinks, and starchy foods or hidden sugars loaded with carbs.

Cutting back on alcohol is still advised, and sticking to the approved list alcohol choices still apply. Remember to only use low-carb or zero soda choices as alcohol mixers and to include a few glasses of water in between alcoholic drinks to avoid dehydration.

Exercise

In Phase 3, you should have a little more energy and your body will be used to the reduced carbohydrate intake. You can increase your exercise routine to what you are comfortable with and fits into your busy schedule. If you find you have to squeeze exercise into your lifestyle, it will start to feel like a chore and you may just give it up altogether.

If you are comfortable with your current routine, up your reps a bit and add 5 to 10 minutes more onto your workout time.

Reaching Your Goal Weight

Upon reaching your goal weight, you will continue on Phase 3 for another four weeks. You will gradually need to increase your carbs by 5 grams at a time. You will need to increase your carb intake amount during these 4 weeks until you reach around 80 grams per day.

Staying on Phase 4 for another four weeks helps you get used to eating at a normal daily carb intake and get used to doing so. You will need to keep a careful eye on your meals, the food you eat, and your weight. Having done this for the past six or more weeks, this should not be that hard.

Carry on making your low-carb meals with some added carbs to pad your intake to your new amount. You can start to add some low-carb baked goods or even increase your snack size. Just remember to keep within your limits and don't fall back into your bad eating habits.

Chapter 6: Phase 4 — Lifestyle Maintenance Phase of the Atkins Diet

Reaching Phase 4 is a huge milestone for you. It means you have reached your goal weight and managed to keep it constant for the past four weeks. Well done!

Phase 4 is the Continuous Maintenance Phase and goes on indefinitely. It is the phase where you transition from the Atkins Diet to the Atkins Lifestyle.

Food List for Phase 4

The following is a list of the acceptable foods that you can enjoy in Phase 4 of the Atkins Diet. Please note that these foods are in addition to the food list laid out in Phase 1, Phase 2, and Phase 3.

Food	Amount	Net Carbs
Alcohol,		
All acceptable alcohol in Phase 2 and 3 apply to Phase 4.		
Beverages, Dairy, Dressings, Eggs, Fats and oils, Fish, Garnishes, Grains, Herbs, Juices, Legumes,		

Meat, Nuts, Poultry, Seeds, Shellfish, Spices, Sweeteners, Starchy Vegetables, and Vegetables		
All acceptable food groups listed in Phase 1, 2, and 3 apply to phase 4.		
Fruit		
All fruit in Phase 2, and 3 apply to Phase 4.		
Pear — medium	1 fruit	21 g
Raisins	1 tablespoon	6.8 g
All legumes in Phase 1 and 2 apply to Phase .4.		

Staying in Control

Phase 4 is all about sticking to your new low-carb eating plan. If you have done so up until now, it should be easy to continue making low-carb food choices. The list of approved foods is not a definitive one; there are loads of low-carb food choices out there. By this phase, you should be on at least 80 grams to 100 grams of carbs per day.

You just need to check the foods you are buying to ensure that they fit into your healthy eating regime. If you do eat high-carb food at a meal or for a snack, make sure you adjust the daily limit around it. There are a lot of low- to no-carb foods that can fill you up for your next meal or snack.

The more adventurous you are with your recipes and food experimentation, the wider your low-carb food choice will become. Try new foods, beverages, and baked goods or treats. In the modern-day, there are a lot of substitutes for the sugary treats and the beverages you love. For instance, use sugar-free low-carb cool drink syrup to make tasty fizzy drinks with club soda or sparkling water. Choose sugar-free maple or caramel syrups to bake with and sugar replacements such as Stevia.

Don't think about the ending of a diet or even keep the word diet, eating plan, or lifestyle in your head. Rather just move with your new flow and keep refining your eating habits as you live your life the low-carb way.

Chapter 7: Atkins for Vegans and Vegetarians

With people opting for plant-based lifestyles, there are now a lot of food substitutes for meat, fish, poultry, and dairy products on the market that are suitable for vegans and vegetarians. The Atkins diet has come a long way since it was first developed and can now be adapted to suit vegan, vegetarian, and pescatarian eating plans.

Some studies have shown that eating a plant-based diet is beneficial to a person's health. Even women who are not vegetarians or vegans will benefit from eating plant-based diets every now and again. They offer nutrient dense meals that do not put a strain on the metabolism as much as consuming meat does.

Health benefits of a plant-based diet include:

- Lowers high blood pressure
- Improve gut function
- Lower cholesterol
- Boost the immunes system
- Reduce inflammation

Vegan

The Atkins Diet can be adjusted to suit the eating preference of vegans. Phase 1 of the Atkins Diet has a lot of restrictions on foods such as nuts, legumes, berries, fruit, and some vegetables. As a vegan, you may find it difficult to start the diet on Phase 1 as you do not eat eggs or dairy products. It is, therefore, recommended that those who follow meat- and dairy-free eating lifestyles start at Phase 2 of the Atkins 20 Diet Plan.

Adapting the Atkins Diet Plan for Vegans

Make the following adjustments to adapt the Atkins diet to a vegan lifestyle:

Start the diet in Phase 2 - Ongoing Weight Loss Phase (OWL)

- Start with 50 g of net carbs per day to lose weight.
- Each week, increase your daily net carb intake by five grams.
- NOTE: Only increase carbs each week if you are losing weight. If not, do not increase your carb limit until you have lost at least one to two pounds.
- Stay in Phase 2 for two weeks.

116

- You can stay in Phase 2 for up to four weeks if you have not come within 10 lbs of your goal weight.
- When you are 10 lbs from your goal weight, progress to Phase 3 — Pre-Maintenance Phase.
- If you want to maintain your weight and only have 10 lbs or less to lose, start the diet in Phase 3.
- Start Phase 3 with 60 grams of net carbs per day.
- In Phase 3, you can increase your net carbs by five grams per week until you reach 80 grams per day, but only increase your carbs if you are losing weight.
- When you have achieved your goal weight, you will stay on Phase 3 without increasing your carb count for another four weeks. This is to make sure you are maintaining your weight at that carb intake level per day.
- If you have maintained your weight for four weeks, you will move into Phase 4, which is the Maintenance and Lifestyle Phase of the diet.
- In Phase 4, you will continue to eat as you did in Phase 3 but you will be able to experiment with more food types as long as

you stick to the recommended daily carb intake.

- The meal plans in Phase 2 in Chapter 4 can be adapted to suit a vegan eating plan.
- The Atkins 100 Diet plan is a great plan for vegans to follow.
- Vegans should take a flax oil supplement.

Foods

The following is a list of foods that are acceptable on the Atkins Diet for vegans; the list is similar to that of Phase 1 and Phase 2 as laid out in the chapters above. For your convenience, I have converged the two lists, taken out the non-vegan foods. I have added some substitute foods for protein and fat replacements. For any beverages that are not listed below, see the lists in the non-vegan Phase 1 to Phase 3 lists in the chapters above.

Food	Amount	Net Carbs
Phase 2 - Ongoing Weight Loss		
Beverages		
Coffee — Decaffeinated or caffeinated (carbs measured for black coffee with no added sugar)	1 cup	0 g

Tea — Regular (carbs measured for black tea with no added sugar) Tea — Herbal (carbs measured for herbal tea with no added sugar)	1 cup	0 g
Water — Sparkling, still, mineral, tap, or spring	1 glass	0 g

Dairy Substitutes

Almond milk — unsweetened, organic	¼ cup	2 g
Coconut cream	1 tablespoon	3.1 g
Coconut milk — unsweetened, organic	¼ cup	3 g
Soya milk	¼ cup	3.5 g

Dressings

Balsamic vinegar	1 tablespoon	2.7 g
Lemon juice	1 tablespoon	1 g
Lime juice	1 tablespoon	1.2 g
Red wine vinegar White wine vinegar	1 tablespoon	0 g

Egg Substitute

Silken tofu — scrambled egg substitute, organic	1 oz	2 g

Vegg — scrambled egg substitute, Vegg — egg yolk substitute	¼ cup	0 g
Vegan Egg	1 large egg	0.6 g

Fats and Oils

Almond butter	¼ cup	0.4 g
Canola oil, Grape seed oil, Olive oil, Sesame oil, Soybean oil, Sunflower oil, Walnut oil	1 tablespoon	0 g
Coconut butter	1 tablespoon	0.8 g
Macadamia butter	1 tablespoon	0.4 g

Fruit

Blackberries	¼ cup	1.6 g
Blueberries	¼ cup	4.5 g
Boysenberries	¼ cup	4.5 g
Cantaloupe	¼ cup	2.9 g
Coconut — unsweetened shredded/fresh	¼ cup	2.3 g
Cranberries	¼ cup	1.9 g

Gooseberries	¼ cup	3.9 g
Honeydew	¼ cup	3.5 g
Raspberries	¼ cup	1.7 g
Herbs		
Basil, Cilantro, Dill, Oregano, Tarragon	1 tablespoon	0 g
Chives	1 tablespoon	0.1 g
Garlic	1 clove	0.9 g
Ginger	1 tablespoon	0.8 g
Parsley	1 tablespoon	0.1 g
Rosemary	1 tablespoon	0.8 g
Sage	1 teaspoon	0.8 g
Juices		
Lemon juice	2 tablespoons	2 g
Lime juice	2 tablespoons	2.4 g
Tomato juice	4 ounces	4 g

Legumes

Black beans	¼ cup	6.5 g
Chickpeas	¼ cup	10.9 g
Great northern beans	¼ cup	10.6 g
Kidney beans	¼ cup	5.9 g
Lima beans	¼ cup	6.1 g
Navy beans	¼ cup	10.1
Pinto beans	¼ cup	6.1 g

Meat Substitutes

Coconut meat	1 ounce	1.7 g
Eggplant	3 ounces	2 g
Portobello mushrooms — medium	2 mushrooms	4 g
Quorn — cutlets	3 ounces	3.7 g
Seitan	3 ounces	0.2 g
Soybeans	¼ cup	0.2 g
Tofu	3 ounces	0.5 g

Nuts		
Almonds	24 nuts	2.2 g
Brazil nuts	6 nuts	1.4 g
Cashews	2 tablespoons	5.1 g
Macadamias	10 nuts	1.4 g
Peanuts	2 tablespoons	3.8 g
Pecans	2 tablespoons	3.8 g
Pine nuts	2 tablespoons	2 g
Pistachios	2 tablespoons	3 g
Walnuts	12 nuts	1.7 g
Seeds		
Chia seeds	2 tablespoons	2 g
Flaxseeds	2 tablespoons	0.2 g

Hemp seeds	2 tablespoons	0.5 g
Poppy seeds	2 tablespoons	2.4 g
Pumpkin seeds	2 tablespoons	2 g
Sesame seeds	2 tablespoons	2 g
Sunflower seeds — hulled	2 tablespoons	1.5 g
Spices		
Black pepper	1 teaspoon	0.9 g
Cayenne pepper	1 teaspoon	0 g
Salt — A dash/pinch of salt (0.4 g) is 155 mg dietary sodium.	1 pinch	0 g
White pepper	1 teaspoon	0.9 g
Sweeteners — Choose a brand that has zero carbs if you can. 1 Packet = 1 tsp		
Saccharine Stevia Sucralose	1 packet	0 to 1 g
Vegetables		
Alfalfa sprouts — Raw	½ cup	0 g
Artichoke — Pickled/marinated	1	1 g

Arugula — Raw	½ cup	0.2 g
Asparagus — Cooked	6 stalks	1.9 g
Avocado — Raw	½	1.3 g
Beet greens — Cooked	½ cup	1.8 g
Bell pepper green — Raw	½ cup	2.2 g
Bell pepper red — Raw	½ cup	3 g
Bell pepper yellow — Raw	½ cup	3 g
Bok choy — Cooked	½ cup	0.4 g
Broccoli — Cooked	½ cup	1.8 g
Broccoli rabe — Cooked	½ cup	1.2 g
Broccolini — Cooked	3	1.9 g
Brussel sprouts — Cooked	½ cup	3.5 g
Button mushroom — Raw	½ cup	0.8 g
Cabbage — Cooked	½ cup	2.7 g
Cauliflower — Cooked	½ cup	1.7 g
Celery — Raw	1 stalk	1 g
Cherry tomato — Raw	10	4.6 g
Chicory greens — Raw	½ cup	0.1 g
Collard greens — Cooked	½ cup	1 g
Cucumber — Raw	½ cup	1.6 g

Dill pickles	1	1 g
Eggplant — Cooked	½ cup	2.3 g
Endive — Raw	½ cup	0.1 g
Escarole — Raw	½ cup	0.1 g
Fennel — Raw	½ cup	1.8 g
Garlic — Minced	2 tablespoons	5.3 g
Green beans — Cooked	½ cup	2.9 g
Kale — Cooked	½ cup	2.4 g
Kohlrabi — Cooked	½ cup	4.6 g
Leeks — Cooked	2 tablespoons	3.4 g
Lettuce — Raw	½ cup	0.5 g
Okra — Cooked	½ cup	1.8 g
Olives black — Raw	5	0.7 g
Olives green — Raw	5	0.1 g
Onion red/white — Raw	2 tablespoons	1.5 g
Portobello mushroom — Cooked	1	2.6 g
Pumpkin — Cooked	½ cup	4.7 g
Radish — Raw	1	0.2 g
Radish (daikon/white) — Raw (grated)	½ cup	1.4 g

Rhubarb — Raw	½ cup	1.8 g
Sauerkraut — Drained	½ cup	1.2 g
Scallion — Raw	½ cup	2.4 g
Shallot — Raw	2 tablespoons	3.4 g
Snow peas — Cooked	½ cup	5.4 g.
Spaghetti squash — Cooked	½ cup	4 g
Spinach — Raw	½ cup	0.2 g
Sprouts/mung beans — Raw	½ cup	2.2 g
Swiss chard — Cooked	½ cup	1.8 g
Tomato small — Raw	1	2.5 g
Turnip greens — Cooked	½ cup	0.6 g
Turnip — Cooked	½ cup	2.4 g
Watercress — Raw	½ cup	0.1 g
Yellow squash — Cooked	½ cup	2.6 g
Zucchini — Cooked	½ cup	1.5 g

Phase 4 Foods

In Phase 4 of the Atkins diet, vegans may start to re-introduce some starchy vegetables along with some whole grain foods.

The foods listed below are to be added to the list above.

Fruit		
All fruit in Phase 1 and 2 apply to Phase 3.		
Apple	½ fruit	7.9 g
Apricot — medium	3 fruit	9.6 g
Banana — small	1 fruit	20.4 g
Cherries	¼ cup	5.3 g
Clementine	1 fruit	7.6 g
Coconut — fresh and unsweetened shredded	½ cup	2.5 g
Dates — fresh	3 fruit	15.8 g
Figs — fresh	1 fruit	4.5 g
Grapes — red	½ cup	13 g
Grapefruit — medium	½ fruit	8.9 g

Guava	½ cup	7.4 g
Kiwi	1 fruit	8.1 g
Mango	½ cup	11.1 g
Orange	½ cup	14.5 g
Papaya	½ cup	6.6 g
Peach — small	1 fruit	10.5 g
Pineapple	½ cup	9.7 g
Plum — medium	1 fruit	6.6 g
Pomegranate seeds	¼ cup	6.4 g
Watermelon	½ cup	5.5 g

Grains		
Barley — cooked	½ cup	19.2 g

Bread — whole wheat	2 slices	20 g
Grits — cooked	½ cup	15.2 g
Millet — cooked	½ cup	19.5 g
Oat bran	2 tablespoons	6.0 g
Oatmeal	⅓ cup	19 g
Pasta — whole wheat and cooked	½ cup	16.6 g
Polenta	2 tablespoons	12.5 g
Quinoa — cooked	¼ cup	8.6 g
Rice — brown and cooked	½ cup	21.2 g
Wheat bran	2 tablespoons	1.6 g
Wheat germ	2 tablespoons	4.9 g

Vegetables — Starchy		
Acorn squash	½ cup	7.6 g

Beets	½ cup	6.8 g
Butternut squash	½ cup	8.5 g
Carrots	½ cup	4 g
Corn	½ cup	14.9 g
Parsnips	½ cup	10.2 g
Peas	½ cup	7 g
Potato — baked, medium	½ potato	13.1 g
Sweet potato — baked, medium	½ potato	9.9 g
Rutabaga	½ cup	5.9 g

Foods to Avoid

Avoid all refined foods, foods with sugar, and starchy vegetables that are not on the acceptable food list. For a more comprehensive list, you can see the foods to avoid in the chapter above for Phase 1.

Vegetarian

Vegetarians can benefit from the Atkins Diet. As per the vegan section above, due to not eating animal proteins, it is advisable for vegetarians to start at Phase 2 of the diet. As pasta and other refined foods are not recommended, excluding these from your diet will help you lose weight.

As you are substituting plant-based proteins for animal proteins, you have to be careful which ones you choose and keep track of the net carbs in them. If you eat eggs, this is a good source to stack your daily protein with.

Adapting the Atkins Diet Plan for Vegetarians

Make the following adjustments to adapt the Atkins diet to a vegetarian lifestyle:

Start the Diet in Phase 2 - Ongoing Weight Loss Phase (OWL)

- Start with 25 to 30 g of net carbs per day to lose weight.
- If you are steadily losing weight, you can increase your net carbs by five grams a day each week.

- Stay in Phase 2 for two weeks or up to four weeks if you have not come within 10 lbs of your goal weight.
- Phase 3 will start when you only have 10 more pounds to lose to reach your goal weight.
- Start Phase 3 with 40 grams of net carbs per day.
- In Phase 3, you can increase your net carbs by five grams per week until you reach 80 grams per day. If you are not losing weight steadily, do not increase your carbs.
- You will stay in Phase 3 until you have reached your goal weight.
- After you have achieved your goal weight, you will stay in Phase 3 for another four weeks to encourage you to keep your new eating habits. This phase is the phase that gets you ready to move onto the lifestyle phase.
- Once you have maintained your goal weight for up to four weeks, you will move onto Phase 4 the Maintenance or Lifestyle Phase.
- The meal plans in Phase 2 in the chapters above can be adapted to suit a vegetarian or pescatarian eating plan.
- As a vegetarian, it is highly recommended that you take either a fish oil or flax oil

supplement to ensure you are getting enough nutrients in your diet.

Foods

You can follow the above vegan acceptable food list, which has a comprehensive list of meat substitutes, vegetables, legumes, fruits, nuts, etc. The list covers acceptable low-carb foods for Phase 2 and Phase 3. Phase 4 is the same as Phase 3, only you will now have the tools and knowledge to experiment with a wider variety of low-carb foods.

For acceptable beverages, including alcohol and dairy products, see the acceptable foods lists for Phase 1, Phase 2, and Phase 3 in the chapters above. You can adjust your food plan by following the tips below:

- If you eat fish and seafood (pescatarian), make sure you use a good portion of these to top up your protein. To get a rich source of Omega-3 fatty acids, try fish such as sardines, salmon, and mackerel.
- Eggs are a good source of protein and can be eaten scrambled, boiled, fried, or in an omelet form.
- Use vegetables such as scallions and herbs to add flavor to your dishes.

- Beans, such as kidney beans, navy beans, lima beans, and soybean are a good source of protein. They are also high in dietary fiber.

- Try meat replacement using vegetables like eggplant. When eggplant is sliced and fried or grilled, it makes a great substitute for bacon. You can use it as a garnish over salads, etc.

- Coconut meat is another good meat replacement and can also be used as a bacon substitute.

- Portobello mushrooms make a tasty replacement for steak. They are a versatile food that is rich in protein and other vital nutrients. You can grill them and use them to add a unique flavor to any salad or dish.

- Replace cow's milk, butter, and creams with nut butter and creams.

- Dairy milk is not allowed on most phases of the Atkins diet and substitutes, such as soy milk, almond, macadamia, and coconut milk, are recommended.

- Make sure you are getting enough fats in your diet.

- Avoid the starchy vegetables that are not on the approved list and eat lots of the vegetables that are on the approved list.

- Eat nuts and seeds to top up on superfoods along with berries and fruit.
- Be careful when eating fruit as there are quite a few carbs in most fruit.

Foods to Avoid

See the chapters above that cover foods to avoid for Phase 1 and Phase 2 as these are the foods that you should stay away from. They are mainly all refined foods, some high-carb starchy vegetables, and baked goods with lots of refined ingredients including sugar. Sweets, soda, and fast foods need to be avoided.

Chapter 8: Living the Atkins Lifestyle

By this chapter, you will have realized that living the Atkins lifestyle is not that difficult. Making healthier choices and watching your carb intake gets easier the more you practice. By the time you have gone onto the Maintenance Phase of the diet, you will already have started to retrain yourself to reach for the lower carb items. Even counting your carbs will soon become second nature to you.

In this chapter, we are going to look at keeping your spirits up, finding your motivation, dealing with slip-ups, and common mistakes to avoid. There are also some general tips for living the Atkins lifestyle and motivational stories.

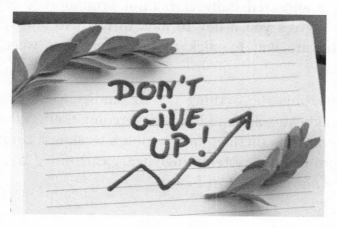

The Challenges Ahead

During your diet, you are going to run into many challenges ahead, most of which will come from yourself.

Slip-Ups and Temptations

It is very easy to get disheartened when dieting. No matter how hard you try, there are going to be times when you slip up or give in to temptation. It is natural and everyone does it. The important thing is how you deal with that slip-up.

Don't get disheartened or stressed out about slipping in and giving into temptation. There is no need to punish yourself. If you know you are going to do it again, rather pick a treat day and work your allocated daily carb limit around that day. This gives you a day to look forward to and will motivate you to stick to achieving your weekly goal.

The important thing is to know what your weaknesses are and how to overcome them. When it comes to dieting, most people's weakness comes from those very tempting sugary carb-filled treats and starchy comfort foods.

The trick to getting around your cravings for these foods is to find something that you can substitute for them. Then train yourself to think about those foods as your comfort treats. For example, if you love ice cream, use a low-carb sweet substitute and make yourself ice blocks. When you crave ice cream, crush the ice blocks in a cup to enjoy instead.

As you progress through the phases in the Atkins diet, you will be able to eat more foods. There are a lot of really tasty baked goods and treats you can make for yourself. Making your own treats is also a lot healthier than buying them from the store. You get to control what goes into the food.

If you find yourself wanting a cake or something sweet while at the store, buy a diet soda to sip on or a bottle of fizzy water. Try not to go to the store when you are hungry. This will increase your cravings for fast foods and treats. Before you go, fill yourself up with a few glasses of water and a low-carb snack. That way the tantalizing smell of the baked goods section won't be as tempting.

Try to keep your slip-ups to a minimum and avoid situations or places you know trigger them.

Some Common Mistakes to Avoid

When you first start out on the diet or even when you are a seasoned Atkins dieter, you can still make mistakes. Here is a list of common mistakes people tend to make on the Atkins Diet:

- **Becoming obsessed with weighing or measuring yourself**

  You should weigh and measure yourself once a week. Make a set day to do this. Only weigh or measure yourself on a different day if you miss your designated one. If you become obsessed with weighing yourself every day, you will start to either lose motivation or revert to starving yourself or over-exercising. Keep calm and trust in the process. As long as you are eating according to plan, you will lose those pounds.

- **Not eating enough vegetables**

  You need to at least eat one or two vegetables on the acceptable food list a day. You need to make sure you are eating at least 15 grams of them a day.

- **Not eating enough protein**

  Your body needs protein and you should be eating at least four ounces a meal. Be careful not to eat too much protein as this could interfere with your weight loss.

- **Trying to avoid fats**

  Lots of people shy away from fats because they have a bad reputation in the nutritional world. There are indeed fats that are bad for you and should be avoided but there are also good ones that are essential for your health. The essential ones are the ones you need to help your body burn fat.

- **Not taking notice of the carbs in foods**

  One of the major pitfalls when it comes to counting carbs is not reading labels or being aware of the hidden sugar in certain foods. Even foods that say they are low-carb or diet foods may have hidden sugars adding to higher carbs. There are many nutritional counter apps that you can quickly look upon if you are in doubt.

- **Not counting carbs correctly**

  Another very common mistake is not counting the net carbs in food. You have to remember to subtract the dietary fiber from the total carbs on a nutrition label.

- **Not keeping a journal**

  Keeping track of the diet is a way to stay motivated, keep yourself on the correct diet path, and take note of things like your progress and foods you like. It is also a great way to help you get in touch with how you feel about yourself. When you start, you may feel you have no confidence, etc. Journaling is a good source of motivation to see how your feelings progress along with your new eating plans

Keeping Motivated

Here are some tips on how to keep yourself motivated to move forward and stay on track:

- Remind yourself that you are doing this for you. To make you feel good about yourself and your lifestyle.

- Don't look at yourself and see the weight that is not there.
- Keep yourself positive by being excited about finding out how much you lost each week.
- Even if you have managed to retain last week's weight loss, that is still a win. Congratulate yourself.
- If you, for some reason, gain a pound or two, don't fret. Try harder next week.
- Don't compare yourself to others. You are you, a unique individual with a body that may have the same sort of shape as another person but it is not the same. There are a lot of factors that make you different from another person.
- Be proud of who you are and what you are accomplishing.
- Don't let negative thoughts creep in. If they do, write them in your journal and tell them you will get back to them. Then write positive thoughts down on the next page that you are addressing today.
- Think of your new lifestyle as a great adventure and have fun with it.

The Atkins Lifestyle and Your Family

When you are on a diet and have a family, it can sometimes mean having to cook two separate meals. Having to cook two separate meals and watch your family eat the foods you enjoy while you eat steamed can quickly make you lose interest in a diet.

By the time you get to this section of the book, you will have seen that the foods you eat on the Atkins diet can be eaten by the entire family. You do, however, have to adjust the serving sizes to ensure your family members are getting enough carbohydrates and nutrients.

Always check with a health care provider, nutritionist, or dietician for your family's exact daily nutrition requirement, especially if they have any pre-existing conditions. The sections below give you an idea of what the recommended daily nutrition intake should be.

Adults

The recommended daily nutritional guideline for an average person consuming 2,000 calories per day:

- 200 g carbohydrates
- 25 to 30 g fiber
- No more than 50 g sugars
- 150 g protein

- No more than 70 g fat
- Less than 20 g saturated fat
- 300 mg cholesterol
- Less than 2,300 mg sodium

Healthy Food Plate for Adults

Picture a dinner plate with a glass on the side.

- **Glass**
  - At least 8 glasses of water
  - Dairy 1 to 2 servings per
  - Juice 1 small glass
- **Plate**
  - Moderate oils such as vegetable oils and fats, and keep trans fats to a minimum.
  - ½ of the plate should contain vegetables and fruits. Stay away or limit starchy vegetables like potatoes, etc.
  - ¼ of the plate should contain whole grains. For example, whole wheat, quinoa, brown pasta, brown rice, steel-cut oats, etc. Limit or cut out refined foods.
  - ¼ of the plate should be protein. For example, meat, fish, poultry, or meat substitutes.

Children

The recommended daily nutritional guideline for children changes with their age.

Daily Recommended Nutrition Guideline for Children 1 to 18							
Age	Sex	Calories	Carbs	Fiber	*Sugar	Protein	*Sodium
1 to 3	B & G	1,000 to 1,200	130 g	19 g	25 g	13 g	1,500 mg
4 to 8	G	1,200 to 1,800	130 g	25 g	25 g	19 g	1,900 mg
4 to 8	B	1,200 to 2,000	130 g	25 g	25 g	19 g	1,900 mg
9 to 13	G	1,400 to 2,200	130 g	26 g	25 g	34 g	2,200 mg
9 to 13	B	1,600 to 2,600	130 g	31 g	25 g	34 g	2,200 mg
14 to 18	G	1,800 to 2,400	130 g	29 g	25 g	46 g	2,300 mg
14 to 18	B	2,000 to 3,200	130 g	38 g	25 g	52 g	2,300 mg

*This is the maximum recommended daily allowance. Try to consume less if possible.

Daily Recommended Nutrition Guideline for Children 1 to 18 based on the recommended calories in the table above.

Age	Sex	Dairy	Fruits	Grains	Protein	Vegies
1 to 3	B & G	2 cups	1-1.5 cups	3-5 oz	2-4 oz	1-1.5 cups
4 to 8	G	2.5 cups	1-1.5 cups	4-6 oz	3-5 oz	1.5-2.5 cups
4 to 8	B	2.5 cups	1-2 cups	4-6 oz	3-5.5 oz	1.5-2.5 cups
9 to 13	G	3 cups	1.5-2 cups	5-7 oz	4-6 oz	1.5-3 cups
9 to 13	B	3 cups	1.5-2 cups	5-9 oz	5-6.5 oz	2-3.5 cups
14 to 18	G	3 cups	1.5-2 cups	6-8 oz	5-6.5 oz	2.5-3 cups
14 to 18	B	3 cups	2-2.5 cups	6-10 oz	5-5.7 oz	2.5-4 cups

Healthy Food Plate for Children

Kids need the same healthy eating food plate breakdown as adults; this includes the fats and oil and beverages.

The table below is a guideline to recommended portions of food groups for kids.

147

Chapter 9: Low-Carb Breakfast Recipes

Here are seven easy-to-make low-carb breakfast recipes.

Please note that the nutritional information is per serving and that the carbohydrates reflect the **net carbs** and **not** the total carbs.

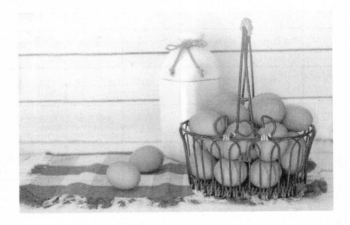

Recipe 1 — Quick and Easy Ham, Mozzarella Cheese, and Mushroom Omelette

This omelet is quick and easy to make. You can microwave the toppings for 1 minute before adding them to the omelet to ensure the ingredients are cooked.

You can add a few more carbs to the recipe by adding to an ingredient or adding another ingredient for diet Phases 3 and 4.

The recipe is suitable for Phase 1 to Phase 4.

Serving Size: 1

Time: 20 minutes

Prep Time: 10 minutes

Cook Time: 10 minutes

Nutritional Facts/Info:

- Calories 311
- Net Carbs 3.4 g
- Fiber 0.5 g
- Sugars 0.9 g
- Fat 21.9 g
- Protein 25.5 g

Ingredients:

- 2 large eggs
- 1 tbsp chopped ham
- 1 tbsp mozzarella cheese — shredded
- 1 tbsp brown mushrooms — chopped
- dash of black pepper
- 1 tsp coconut oil

Directions:

1. In a mixing bowl, beat eggs with a dash of black pepper.
2. Heat coconut oil in an omelet pan.
3. Pour the egg mixture into the pan.
4. Allow to cook for 1 minute, or until the omelet is cooked through.
5. Flip with a spatula and add the chopped ham, chopped mushrooms, and shredded cheese.
6. Flavor with a dash of black pepper.
7. Flip the one half of the omelet to cover the ingredients.
8. Flip the folded omelet and cook for 30 seconds to 1 minute.
9. Flip the folded omelet onto the other side for another 30 seconds.

10. Remove the pan from the heat and dish the omelet onto a breakfast plate.

Recipe 2 — Green Bell Pepper Stuffed With Steak and Baby Spinach

Bell peppers are a good source of iron. They make a delicious breakfast for a great start to the day.

If you are using this recipe for Phase 2 and up, you can add cream or cottage cheese to it to increase the net carbs.

The recipe is suitable for Phase 1 to Phase 4.

Serving Size: 1

Time: 25 minutes

Prep Time: 10 minutes

Cook Time: 15 minutes

Nutritional Facts/Info:

- Calories 162
- Net Carbs 3.9 g
- Fiber 2.2 g
- Sugars 3 g
- Fat 7.2 g
- Protein 18.7 g

Ingredients:

- 1.7 oz steak — cut into strips
- 1 medium green bell pepper — whole
- 1 tbsp brown mushrooms — diced
- 2 tbsp baby spinach leaves — shredded
- ¼ tsp garlic — crushed
- 1 tsp coconut oil or vegetable oil
- dash of black pepper

Directions:

1. In a skillet, heat the coconut or vegetable oil over medium heat.
2. Cook the steak to your cooking preference.
3. Add the crushed garlic, mushrooms, and spinach; sauté for 1 to 2 minutes. Add these ingredients 1 to 2 minutes before the steak is cooked.
4. Remove the ingredients from the pan and put on a plate to cool slightly.
5. Cut the top off the bell pepper and remove the seeds.
6. Using the same skillet you cooked the steak in, heat the green pepper to slightly soften it. Do not overcook it or burn it.
7. Remove the bell pepper from the skillet and place it on a plate.
8. Stuff the pepper with the steak mixture and serve.

Recipe 3 — Breakfast Blueberry Muffins

These muffins are cooked in the microwave and take only 15 minutes to make. They are great for an on-the-go breakfast.

The recipe is Suitable for Phase 2 to Phase 4.

Serving Size: 1

Time: 12 minutes

Prep Time: 10 minutes

Cook Time: 2 minutes

Nutritional Facts/Info:

- Calories 217
- Net Carbs 7.3 g
- Fiber 0.9 g
- Sugars 4.2g
- Fat 13.3 g
- Protein 15.8 g

Ingredients:

- 1 egg — at room temperature
- 3 tbsp blueberries — fresh or unsweetened if frozen
- ¼ tsp sesame seeds

- 2 tbsp whey protein powder — vanilla
- 2 tbsp cream cheese
- dash of nutmeg
- ¼ tsp baking powder
- ¼ tsp vanilla extract

Directions:

1. Whisk together the cream cheese and egg in a mixing bowl.
2. Add the baking powder, nutmeg, egg, vanilla extract, and whey protein powder.
3. Whisk together until the mixture is well mixed.
4. Mix in the sesame seeds and blueberries.
5. Pour the mixture into a microwavable mug.
6. Place the mixture in the mug into the microwave for 1 minute.
7. After a minute, test to see if the muffin is done by gently inserting a clean knife or skewers into the middle of it.
8. If the knife or skewer comes out clean, the muffin is done. If not, heat it for another 10 to 15 seconds at a time until the knife comes out clean when inserted into the middle.
9. Tip the muffin onto a cooling rack or plate to cool for a few seconds before eating it.

Recipe 4 — Smoked Salmon, Dill, and Avocado with Poached Egg

In phase 1, you can only use ½ the avocado, but as you progress to the next phase, you can use both halves of the avocado to increase the carb count. Avocados are a great source of good fats, high in fiber, and good for controlling cholesterol.

The recipe is Suitable for Phase 1 to Phase 4.

Serving Size: 1

Time: 15 minutes

Prep Time: 10 minutes

Cook Time: 5 minutes

Nutritional Facts/Info:

- Calories 310
- Net Carbs 3.5 g
- Fiber 7.3 g
- Sugars 0.9 g
- Fat 26.1 g
- Protein 12 g

Ingredients:

- 1 large egg
- 1 tbsp smoked salmon — shredded
- ½ avocado
- 3 cherry tomatoes — halved
- 1 tsp mozzarella cheese — shredded
- ¼ tsp dill
- dash of chili pepper (optional)
- dash of ground black pepper

Directions:

1. Poach the egg.
2. Place the halved cherry tomatoes in the halved avocado.
3. Place ½ the dill, ½ the mozzarella, and ½ the smoked salmon on top of the tomatoes.
4. Place the poached egg on top of the halved avocado.
5. Add the leftover dill, smoked salmon, and mozzarella on top of the poached egg.
6. Sprinkle a dash of chili pepper and freshly ground black pepper to taste.

Recipe 5 — Berry Coconut Breakfast Parfait

This parfait makes a great sweet and tangy breakfast meal. You can add a dash of cayenne pepper to give it some spice. If you feel you need a bit more sweetness, you can add another tsp of sweetener.

The recipe is Suitable for Phase 2 to Phase 4.

Serving Size: 1

Time: 15 minutes

Prep Time: 15 minutes

Cook Time: N/A

Nutritional Facts/Info:

- Calories 204
- Net Carbs 6.9 g
- Fiber 3.4 g
- Sugars 4.9 g
- Fat 16 g
- Protein 6.6 g

Ingredients:

- 1 tbsp blackberries — fresh, unsweetened if frozen
- 1 tbsp raspberries — fresh, unsweetened if frozen
- 2 medium strawberries — halved
- ¼ cup fresh coconut meat — shredded, unsweetened if bought shredded
- ¼ cup cream — heavy
- ¼ cup Greek yogurt — fat-free
- 2 tsp Stevia (2 x 1 g sachets) — you can use any of the acceptable sweeteners
- ½ tsp vanilla extract

Directions:

1. In a large mixing bowl, blend the yogurt, cream, vanilla, and 1 tsp of Stevia.
2. Blend the mixture with a whisk or blender on medium until mixture forms soft peaks.
3. Cut the blackberries and raspberries into halves.
4. Place ½ of the cut blackberries and ½ of the cut raspberries into a small mixing bowl.
5. Purée the berries in the small mixing bowl.
6. Fold the remaining blackberries and raspberries into the purée.

7. Gently mix 1 tsp (1 sachet) of Stevia into the pure mixture.
8. If you are using fresh coconut meat, chop it into bite-sized chunks.
9. In a parfait glass or breakfast bowl:
    o Scoop in 1 tbsp yogurt/cream mixture.
    o Top the yogurt with a sprinkling of coconut.
    o Top the yogurt with 1 tbsp berry purée mixture.
    o Top the berry purée with a sprinkling of coconut.
    o Continue layering the parfait until both mixtures are finished
    o The parfait works well if you end it with the yogurt mixture.
    o Leave enough coconut to sprinkle on the top of the parfait.
10. Top the parfait with the 2 halved fresh strawberries.

Recipe 6 — *Goat Cheese, Asparagus, and Turkey Scramble*

You can add 1 tbsp chopped tomato or ½ tsp roasted sesame seeds to this recipe from Phase 2 to Phase 4.

The recipe is Suitable for Phase 1 to Phase 4.

Serving Size: 1

Time: 25 minutes

Prep Time: 10 minutes

Cook Time: 15 minutes

Nutritional Facts/Info:

- Calories 273
- Net Carbs 1.9 g
- Fiber 1.2 g
- Sugars 1.9 g
- Fat 17.7 g
- Protein 25.5 g

Ingredients:

- 2 eggs
- 3 medium asparagus spears
- 1 oz turkey — shredded
- 1 oz goat cheese
- 1 tsp basil — shredded
- 1 tsp coconut or vegetable oil
- dash of black or red pepper to tastes

Directions:

1. In a mixing bowl, beat the eggs.
2. Add a dash of black pepper.
3. Chop the asparagus spears in bite-sized chunks.
4. Heat the oil in a skillet over medium heat.
5. Add the beaten eggs and stir in the asparagus.
6. When the eggs are done, remove them from the heat.
7. Add the turkey, goat cheese, and basil.
8. Add a dash of black pepper to taste and serve.

Recipe 7 — Pumpkin, Almond, and Vanilla Whey Protein Sour Cream Pancakes

You can enjoy these delicious pumpkin pancakes with a dollop of sour cream.

The nutritional information is calculated per pancake.

The recipe is Suitable for Phase 2 to Phase 4.

Serving Size: 6 pancakes

Time: 20 minutes

Prep Time: 10 minutes

Cook Time: 10 minutes

Nutritional Facts/Info:

- Calories 221
- Net Carbs 3.9 g
- Fiber 1.6 g
- Sugars 1.8 g
- Fat 12.4 g
- Protein 21.9 g

Ingredients:

- 4 large eggs — at room temperature
- ½ cup almond flour — blanched
- 1 tsp baking powder
- 4 oz whey protein — vanilla
- ½ cup cooked pumpkin — mashed
- ¼ low-fat plain cottage cheese — chunky
- ½ tsp pumpkin spice
- 3 tbsp sour cream
- 1 tbsp coconut or vegetable oil

Directions:

1. Beat the eggs in a mixing bowl.
2. In another mixing bowl, mix almond flour, cooked pumpkin, baking powder, and cottage cheese.
3. Whisk the beaten eggs into the almond flour mixture until the mixture is light and fluffy.
4. Add the pumpkin spice and stir it into the mixture well.
5. Lightly grease a large non-stick pan with coconut or vegetable oil. You can use butter to grease the pan as it will not add to the carbohydrate count. It does slightly increase the fat and protein count.

6. Heat the greased non-stick pan over a hot plate.

7. Each pancake takes approximately 3 tablespoons (¼ cup) of the mixture.

8. Using either a cup or tablespoon, scoop the mixture onto the heated non-stick pan.

9. You should be able to get at least 3 pancakes in a large pan at a time.

10. Turn the pancakes after about 2 minutes or when the pancake is firm.

11. Once the second side is done, remove the pancake from the heat.

12. Light grease and heat the pan once again.

13. Repeat steps 7 to 11 until you have used all the pancake batter.

14. Serve pancakes with a dollop (1 tsp) of whipped sour cream.

Chapter 10: Low-Carb Lunch Recipes

Here are seven easy-to-make low-carb lunch recipes.

Please note that the nutritional information is per serving and that the carbohydrates reflect the **net carbs** and **not** the total carbs.

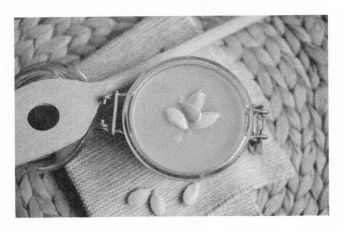

Recipe 8 — Portobello Mushrooms Topped With Red Bell Pepper, Zucchini, and Swiss Cheese

You can leave off the cheese for a dairy-free meal choice in phase 1. In phase 2, you can add ½ tbsp crushed cashews, which will add 1.3 g of net carbs to the recipe.

The recipe is suitable for Phase 1 to Phase 4.

Serving Size: 1

Time: 20 minutes

Prep Time: 10 minutes

Cook Time: 10 minutes

Nutritional Facts/Info:

- Calories 158
- Net Carbs 3.3 g
- Fiber 0.3 g
- Sugars 1 g
- Fat 11.7 g
- Protein 8.8 g

Ingredients:

- 1 large portobello mushroom
- 1 tbsp green bell pepper — finely chopped
- 1 tbsp zucchini — finely chopped
- 1 slice of Swiss cheese
- ¼ tsp butter
- ¼ tsp garlic — crushed
- cayenne pepper to taste

Directions:

1. Use ½ tsp butter to spread on the underside of the mushroom.
2. Spread the crushed garlic over the butter.
3. Heat the grill and place the portobello mushroom on the grill.
4. Grill for 3 to 5 minutes; the mushroom should be slightly tender.
5. Heat the chopped zucchini and green pepper with the leftover butter in the microwave for 1 minute.
6. Add a dash of cayenne pepper to the mix and stir it in well.
7. Place the heated zucchini and green pepper on the portobello mushroom.
8. Break the Swiss cheese and layer it over the zucchini and green pepper.
9. Place the portobello mushroom in the grill until the cheese has melted.

10. Remove from the grill when the cheese is slightly browned and it will be ready to serve.
11. If you are adding crushed cashews, add the cashews before you serve the mushroom.

Recipe 9 — Artichoke and Sesame Seed Salad

Try something different with this artichoke salad sprinkled with sesame seeds, pine nuts, watercress, and goat cheese.

The recipe is suitable for Phase 2 to Phase 4.

Serving Size: 1

Time: 10 minutes

Prep Time: 10 minutes

Cook Time: N/A

Nutritional Facts/Info:

- Calories 132
- Net Carbs 2.1 g
- Fiber 2 g
- Sugars 4.1 g
- Fat 12.3 g
- Protein 2.8 g

Ingredients:

- ½ Artichoke heart — marinated
- 2 tbsp cup watercress — chopped
- 1 tsp fresh basil — chopped
- 1 tsp roasted sesame seeds

- 1 tsp pine nuts
- 1 tbsp goat cheese — crumbled
- 1 tsp balsamic vinegar
- 1 tsp virgin olive oil
- 1 tbsp red wine vinegar
- 1 tsp Stevia or sweetener on the approved foods list

Directions:

1. Chop artichoke hearts into bite-sized pieces and place them in a medium-sized salad bowl.
2. Add chopped watercress, basil, sesame seeds, and pine nuts.
3. Crumble the goat cheese over the salad.
4. In a jar, mix the virgin olive oil, balsamic vinegar, red wine vinegar, and Stevia.
5. Shake the olive mixture well and drizzle over the artichoke salad.

Recipe 10 — Steak, Spinach, Avocado, and Brown Mushroom Bowl

This is a nice meal to eat either hot or cold. If you are going to eat it cold, you will only have to cook the steak. Use baby spinach leaves instead of regular spinach and do not cook the mushrooms.

To use it as a meal for Phase 2 and up, you can add some nuts, seeds, and cheese of your choice. Feta, goat cheese, or blue cheese complements this dish nicely.

You can leave off the mayonnaise and garlic sauce.

The recipe is suitable for Phase 1 to Phase 4.

Serving Size: 1

Time: 25 minutes

Prep Time: 10 minutes

Cook Time: 15 minutes

Nutritional Facts/Info:

- Calories 296
- Net Carbs 7.3 g
- Fiber 1.3 g
- Sugars 2.8 g

- Fat 19.4 g
- Protein 22.3 g

Ingredients:

- 2 oz steak — cut into strips
- ¼ spinach
- ¼ cup brown mushrooms — halved
- ½ avocado — Hass
- ¼ tsp garlic — crushed
- ¼ tsp mustard powder
- 1 tbsp mayonnaise
- black to taste
- dash of cayenne pepper
- 2 tsp coconut oil or vegetable oil

Directions:

1. In a small mixing bowl, mix together the mayonnaise, mustard powder, garlic, and a dash of cayenne pepper.
2. Cover the mayonnaise mixture and put it into the refrigerator.
3. Heat coconut or vegetable oil in a large skillet.
4. Add the steak strips and sear for 1 to 2 minutes.
5. Add the mushroom and allow to cook with the steak for 1 to 2 minutes.
6. Rip the spinach into large shreds and add to the skillet.
7. Flavor with black pepper to taste.
8. Remove when the steak is cooked to your liking.
9. The spinach and the mushrooms should be soft and not overcooked.
10. Add the steak mixture into a bowl.
11. Drizzle with the mayonnaise mixture.
12. Slice the avocado half into strips and add it to the top of the steak mixture.

Recipe 11 — Salmon, Avocado, and Feta Green Leaf Salad

Salmon and feta cheese make a mouthwatering combination when paired in a salad.

If you are using this salad in Phase 2 to Phase 4, add 1 tbsp blackberries and some pine nuts.

The recipe is suitable for Phase 1 to Phase 4.

Serving Size: 1

Time: 10 minutes

Prep Time: 10 minutes

Cook Time: N/A

Nutritional Facts/Info:

- Calories 163
- Net Carbs 1.3 g
- Fiber 0.3 g
- Sugars 1 g
- Fat 11.2 g
- Protein 13.4 g

Ingredients:

- 2 oz smoked salmon — shredded
- 2 tbsp feta cheese — crumbled
- ¼ cup lettuce — shredded
- ¼ cup baby spinach — shredded
- 2 tbsp watercress — shredded
- 1 tbsp white wine vinegar
- 1 tsp olive oil
- 1 tsp Stevia or sweetener on the approved list

Directions:

1. In a bowl, mix together the white wine vinegar, olive oil, and Stevia.
2. Shake the dress well so all the mixture combines.
3. In a salad bowl, mix together the lettuce, baby spinach, and watercress.
4. Add the smoked salmon and gently work it into the salad leaves.
5. Add the feta cheese.
6. Drizzle with the olive oil and vinegar salad dressing.

Recipe 12 — Hearty Cream of Asparagus Soup

This recipe can be enjoyed all year long. It can be used as a lunch or dinner recipe and can be complemented with pumpkin seeds for Phase 2 of the Atkins diet.

The recipe is suitable for Phase 1 to Phase 4.

Serving Size: 4 portions

Time: 55 minutes

Prep Time: 25 minutes

Cook Time: 30 minutes

Nutritional Facts/Info:

- Calories 93
- Net Carbs 4.7 g
- Fiber 2.8 g
- Sugars 3.9 g
- Fat 5 g
- Protein 6 g

Ingredients:

- 1 lb asparagus —chopped
- 2 celery stalks — chopped
- ½ red onion — chopped into large chunks
- 21.5 oz vegetable broth
- ½ cup cream — heavy
- dash of salt
- black pepper to taste
- 2 tsp coconut oil or vegetable oil

Directions:

1. In a large saucepan, heat the coconut or vegetable oil.
2. Place the onions into the saucepan and cook until soft and glassy.
3. Add the celery and asparagus to the saucepan.
4. Add the salt and slowly pour in the vegetable broth.
5. Bring the mixture to a slow boil, then turn the heat down to a simmer.
6. Cover the saucepan and allow the soup to simmer gently for 20 minutes.
7. After 20 minutes, remove the soup from the stove and allow it to cool down for 10 minutes.

8. When the soup has cooled down to warm, pour it into a blender and purée.
9. When the soup is smooth, pour it back into the saucepan, add the cream, some salt, and pepper to taste.
10. Heat on medium heat for another 10 minutes until the soup is piping hot.
11. Remove from the stove, add to soup bowls, and enjoy.

Recipe 13 — *Low-Carb Cheesy Sausage and Mushroom Pizza*

When you move to Phase 2 and 3, you can enjoy more foods, like low-carb pizza with flour basses. This is a pizza that you can enjoy from Phase 1 and has a cauliflower base.

This recipe can also be used as a dinner recipe.

The recipe is suitable for Phase 1 to Phase 4.

Serving Size: 4 pieces of pizza

Time: 55 minutes

Prep Time: 10 minutes

Cook Time: 45 minutes

Nutritional Facts/Info:

- Calories 53
- Net Carbs 4.6 g
- Fiber 1.5 g
- Sugars 3 g
- Fat 2.5 g
- Protein 2.8 g

Ingredients:

- 1 egg
- ½ small white onion — chopped
- ½ red bell pepper — chopped
- 1 cauliflower head — medium (must be equivalent to 3 cups)
- 1 tbsp pitted sliced black olives
- 1 tbsp pitted sliced green olives
- 1 cup mozzarella cheese — shredded
- 1 cup Parmesan cheese — shredded
- 2 tbsp tomato paste — unsweetened, organic
- ¼ tsp cayenne pepper
- ¼ tsp garlic salt
- ¼ tsp Italian spice

Directions:

1. Preheat the oven to 435° F.
2. Boil the cauliflower on the stove or in the microwave until it is soft enough to mash.
3. When the cauliflower is cooked, let it cool down for 10 to 15 minutes.
4. When the cauliflower is cool, squeeze out any excess water from the vegetable.
5. Mash the base together with the Parmesan cheese.

6. Fold the egg into the mixture and add the Italian spice, the cayenne pepper, and garlic salt.
7. Make the mixture into a tight ball.
8. Cut parchment paper to fit a 9-inch round pizza or pie dish.
9. Place the parchment in the round dish.
10. Put the cauliflower dough into the dish and form it into a round pizza base. It should be about ¼ inch thick.
11. Place the cauliflower pizza base into the pre-heated oven for 18 to 20 minutes. Turn the base half-way through the baking process to ensure both sides cook evenly.
12. When the crust is a nice golden brown, remove it from the oven and let it cool for five minutes.
13. When the crust is cool enough to touch, spread the tomato paste on the base.
14. Top with the finely chopped onion, bell pepper, and olives.
15. Spread the mozzarella cheese over the top.
16. Place the pizza back into the oven to bake for another 8 to 10 minutes.
17. When the pizza is cooked through, remove it from the oven and let it cool for 2 to 5 minutes.
18. Cut the pizza into 4 slices and serve.

Recipe 14 — Portobello Chicken Burger With Feta and Shallots

You can swap the chicken out for beef or turkey in this recipe.

From Phase 2, you can add 1 slice of tomato (0.4 g net carbs) to the burger and ½ a dill pickle (0.3 g net carbs). Remember to keep an eye on your carb count.

The recipe is suitable for Phase 1 to Phase 4.

Serving Size: 1

Time: 25 minutes

Prep Time: 10 minutes

Cook Time: 15 minutes

Nutritional Facts/Info:

- Calories 132
- Net Carbs 1.8 g
- Fiber 0.5 g
- Sugars 0.8 g
- Fat 7.5 g
- Protein 13.8 g

Ingredients:

- 2 oz chicken — minced
- 2 medium portobello mushrooms — remove the stalk
- 1 tsp shallots — chopped
- 2 tbsp feta cheese — crumbled
- black pepper to taste
- 1 tsp coconut oil or vegetable oil

Directions:

1. Add the chopped shallots, 1 tbsp crumbled feta cheese, and pepper to taste to the minced chicken.
2. Work the chicken into a burger patty shape.
3. In a skillet, heat the coconut or vegetable oil.
4. Cook the chicken burger patty until it is cooked through.
5. Top each of the portobello mushrooms with ½ tbsp feta cheese.
6. Heat the grill and add the two portobello mushrooms.
7. Grill the mushrooms until warm and slightly soft.
8. Remove the mushrooms from the grill.

9. Place the chicken burger patty on one of the mushrooms.
10. Cover the top of the burger with the other mushroom.

Chapter 11: Low-Carb Dinner Recipes

Here are 7 easy-to-make low-carb dinner recipes.

Please note that the nutritional information is per serving and that the carbohydrates reflect the **net carbs** and **not** the total carbs.

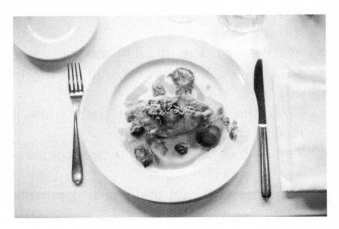

Recipe 15 — *Beef Stroganoff on a Bed of Green Beans*

This is a simple and easy-to-cook low-carb beef stroganoff that is complemented by the taste of the green beans.

The recipe is suitable for Phase 2 to Phase 4.

Serving Size: 2

Time: 30 minutes

Prep Time: 10 minutes

Cook Time: 20 minutes

Nutritional Facts/Info:

- Calories 167
- Net Carbs 7.5 g
- Fiber 3.2 g
- Sugars 3 g
- Fat 7.6 g
- Protein 3 g

Ingredients:

- 2 oz stir fry beef
- 1 cup brown mushrooms — halved
- ½ white onion — chopped
- 1 cup green beans — fresh and halved
- ½ cup beef broth
- ¼ glass of red wine
- 2 tbsp cream — soured
- salt and black pepper to taste
- 1 tsp mustard powder
- 1 tbsp coconut or vegetable oil
- ½ tbsp of butter — unsalted

Directions:

1. Heat the oil in a saucepan on medium heat.
2. Brown the meat and onion.
3. When the meat has been seared and the onion is glassy, remove the ingredients from the saucepan. Put them to one side.
4. Using the same saucepan, melt the butter, add the mushrooms, and sauté until they are soft but still firm.
5. Add the wine and beef broth to the mushrooms.
6. Allow the mixture to simmer on medium heat for 8 to 10 minutes.

7. While the mixture is simmering, cook the green beans in a saucepan of water over medium heat.

8. When the beans are soft but firm, remove from the stove and drain off excess water.

9. Add a bit of black pepper to taste and put them in a warmer drawer.

10. After 8 to 10 minutes, add the meat mixture and stir in well.

11. Slowly pour in the sour cream, stirring as you pour it into the mixture.

12. Turn the stove down to a heat that allows the stroganoff to simmer gently.

13. Allow the mixture to simmer for a further 3 to 5 minutes.

14. When the mixture is cooked, remove from the heat.

15. Add salt and pepper to taste.

16. Dish the green beans into two bowls.

17. Top the green beans with the beef stroganoff and serve while hot.

Recipe 16 — Fillet Medallions With Blackberry, Feta, and Spinach Salad

In Phase 2 of the Atkins diet, you can start to enjoy fruits and berries. This steak salad bursts with flavor with the mix of blackberries and feta.

The recipe is suitable for Phase 2 to Phase 4.

Serving Size: 1

Time: 25 minutes

Prep Time: 10 minutes

Cook Time: 15 minutes

Nutritional Facts/Info:

- Calories 361
- Net Carbs 6.3 g
- Fiber 2 g
- Sugars 3 g
- Fat 28.7 g
- Protein 19.6 g

Ingredients:

- 2 oz beef fillet steak — cut into 1-inch medallions
- 2 tbsp blackberries — halved
- ¼ baby spinach leaves — shredded
- 2 tbsp arugula
- 2 tbsp feta cheese — crumbled
- 1 tbsp fresh basil
- 1 tsp roasted sesame seeds (optional)
- 1 tbsp mayonnaise
- 1 tsp mustard powder
- 1 tsp stevia or sweetener of your choice on the approved foods list
- ½ tsp tomato sauce
- 2 tsp coconut oil or vegetable oil

Directions:

1. In a large skillet, heat the coconut or vegetable oil
2. Cook the fillet medallions to your liking.
3. When the steak is cooked, remove it from the heat and put it to one side to cool.
4. In a salad bowl, mix the arugula, baby spinach leaves, and basil.
5. In a jar or jug, mix together the mayonnaise, mustard powder, tomato

sauce, and Stevia. You can add a dash of white wine vinegar to give it an extra tang and make the mixture a little runny.

6. When the steak has cooled down, mix it into the salad bowl.

7. Add the blackberries, sesame seeds, and crumbled feta cheese.

8. Drizzle the mayonnaise dressing over it — try the salad with just a bit of pepper first as you may not like the mayonnaise dressing mix with the berries.

Recipe 17 — Lamb Chops With Cauliflower Mash

Lamb chops work well with mashed cauliflower and a bit of Dijon mustard.

The recipe is suitable for Phase 1 to Phase 4.

Serving Size: 1

Time: 25 minutes

Prep Time: 10 minutes

Cook Time: 15 minutes

Nutritional Facts/Info:

- Calories 478
- Net Carbs 5.6 g
- Fiber 6.2 g
- Sugars 1.2 g
- Fat 37.1 g
- Protein 26.5 g

Ingredients:

- 1 lamb chop
- ½ cup cauliflower
- 4 cherry tomatoes — halved
- ¼ cup brown mushrooms — halved

- ¼ avocado
- 2 tsp coconut oil
- 2 tsp Dijon mustard
- 2 tsp unsalted butter
- 1 tsp rosemary — fresh (crushed) or dried
- 1 ¼ tsp salt
- 1 ¼ tsp black pepper

Directions:

1. Boil the cauliflower in a saucepan of water until soft enough to mash.
2. When the cauliflower is done, drain off all excess water.
3. Add ¼ tsp of salt and ¼ black pepper to flavor. You do not have to use all of the designated amounts of salt or pepper; season to your taste.
4. While the cauliflower is cooking, rub each of the lamb chops with a bit of coconut oil and Dijon mustard.
5. Mix 1 tsp black pepper, 1 tsp salt, and 1 tsp rosemary on a dinner plate.
6. Dip the lamb chop rubbed with coconut oil onto the rosemary mix. Do both sides of the chop to coat them with the rosemary mix.
7. Put the lamb chop into a grilling/baking dish and place under the grill until cooked to your liking.

8. About 2 minutes before the chop is ready to come off the grill, add the mushrooms and cherry tomatoes.
9. Dish the cauliflower mash onto a plate.
10. Top the cauliflower mash with the lamb chop, grilled tomato, and mushrooms.
11. Slice the ¼ avocado in long medium-thick slices and serve with the dish.

Recipe 18 — *Cauliflower and Minced Beef Fritters*

You can use cauliflower with minced beef to make tasty beef fritters.

The recipe is suitable for Phase 2 to Phase 4.

Serving Size: 6 fritters

Time: 25 minutes

Prep Time: 10 minutes

Cook Time: 15 minutes

Nutritional Facts/Info:

- Calories 142
- Net Carbs 2 g
- Fiber 1.2 g
- Sugars 0.4 g
- Fat 9.4 g
- Protein 12.2 g

Ingredients:

- 1 egg
- 3 oz ground beef
- ½ cup cauliflower — mashed
- 1 tbsp shallots — finely chopped

- 1 cup iceberg lettuce — shredded
- 2 tbsp fresh basil — shredded
- ¼ cup arugula — shredded
- 2 tbsp almond flour — blanched
- 2 tsp coconut oil or vegetable oil
- 1 tsp mixed herb spice
- dash of black pepper to taste

Directions:

1. Cook and mash the cauliflower.
2. In a mixing bowl, mix the ground beef and cauliflower mash.
3. Fold the egg into the ground beef and cauliflower mixture.
4. Add the finely chopped shallots to the ground beef and cauliflower mixture.
5. Sift in the almond flour a bit at a time to firm the mixture.
6. Add the mixed herb spice and pepper to taste.
7. Divide the mixture up into 4 to 6 balls and flatten into 1.4-inch thick fritter rounds.
8. Heat the coconut oil in a skillet.
9. You should be able to cook at least 3 fritters at a time in the skillet.
10. When they are cooked, dish up onto a plate and serve on a bed of crisp shredded lettuce, arugula, and basil leaves.

Recipe 19 — *Vegetable Lamb Stew*

This hearty beef stew can be enjoyed as a dinner or lunch recipe.

The recipe is suitable for Phase 2 to Phase 4.

Serving Size: 2

Time: 1 hour and 20 minutes

Prep Time: 20 minutes

Cook Time: 1 hour

Nutritional Facts/Info:

- Calories 476
- Net Carbs 5.6 g
- Fiber 1.9 g
- Sugars 3.6 g
- Fat 22 g
- Protein 58.9 g

Ingredients:

- 14 oz lamb — cubed
- ¼ cup turnip
- ¼ cup cauliflower
- ¼ brussels sprouts
- 1 white onion — chopped

- 1 garlic clove — crushed
- 6.7 fl. oz vegetable broth
- 2 tsp fresh basil
- 2 tbsp vegetable oil
- pepper to taste

Directions:

1. Heat 1 tsp of vegetable oil in a medium pot over medium heat.
2. Add chopped onions and cook until glassy.
3. Remove onions from the pot and put them to one side.
4. Add 1 tsp of vegetable oil to the pot you removed the onions from.
5. Brown lamb cubes in the heated oil.
6. Add the chopped turnip, cauliflower, and brussels sprouts.
7. Add the vegetable stock and cooked onions to the ingredients in the pot.
8. Bring to a boil and then turn the heat down to allow the stew to simmer.
9. Add the crushed garlic clove, basil, and season to taste.
10. Cover the stew and allow it to simmer gently for 1 hour or until the meat and vegetables are soft.
11. Dish into bowls and serve hot.

Recipe 20 — Simple Vegetable Beef Chili

This warm chili can be adjusted to suit how spicy you want it to be. For this recipe, the chili is mild to medium spiced.

The recipe is suitable for Phase 1 to Phase 4.

Serving Size: 2

Time: 35 minutes

Prep Time: 10 minutes

Cook Time: 25 minutes

Nutritional Facts/Info:

- Calories 436
- Net Carbs 3.9 g
- Fiber 5 g
- Sugars 4.4 g
- Fat 24 g
- Protein 30 g

Ingredients:

- 3 oz ground beef
- 1 cup brown mushrooms — halved
- ¼ cup zucchini — chopped into bite-sized chunks

- ¼ cup pumpkin — bite-sized cubes
- 1 tsp garlic — crushed
- 2 tbsp cream — heavy
- ¼ cup beef broth
- 2 tsp chili powder — mild to medium
- 1 tsp black pepper
- 1 tsp mixed herbs spice
- 1 tsp coconut oil or vegetable oil

Directions:

1. On the stove or in the microwave, cook the chopped zucchini until it is firm but starting to get soft.
2. Drain all excess water off the zucchini once it is done and put it to one side.
3. On the stove or in the microwave, cook the cubed pumpkin until it is firm but starting to get soft.
4. Drain all the excess water off the pumpkin once it is done and put it to one side.
5. Heat oil in a saucepan.
6. Add ground beef and crushed garlic.
7. Flavor the ground beef with mixed herbs and black pepper.
8. When the ground beef is browned, add the mushrooms, semi-cooked zucchini, and pumpkin.
9. Add the beef broth, chili powder, and pepper to taste.

10. Bring the mixture to a boil stirring it regularly.
11. Turn the chili down to low heat and allow it to simmer for 10 minutes to allow the flavor to set and the vegetable to soften.
12. After 10 minute stir in the cream.
13. Allow the mixture to simmer for a further 5 minutes before removing from heat.
14. Dish into bowls and serve piping hot.

Recipe 21 — Chicken Breast Stuffed With Goat Cheese and Asparagus

This dish can be used for a lunch recipe as well. It can be served hot or cold.

You do not have to use the mustard mayonnaise sauce if you do not wish to.

The recipe is suitable for Phase 1 to Phase 4.

Serving Size: 2

Time: 53 minutes

Prep Time: 15 minutes

Cook Time: 38 minutes

Nutritional Facts/Info:

- Calories 296
- Net Carbs 3 g
- Fiber 1.5 g
- Sugars 2 g
- Fat 14.3 g
- Protein 36.2 g

Ingredients:

- 2 x 4 oz lean chicken breasts
- 6 large asparagus stalks — halved

- ¼ brown mushrooms — halved
- 1 tsp dill — finely chopped
- 1 tbsp goat cheese — semi-soft
- ¼ tsp garlic — crushed
- 1 tsp butter
- 2 tsp mayonnaise
- cayenne or black pepper to taste
- ¼ tsp mustard powder

Directions:

1. Preheat the oven to 350° F.
2. Cut each chicken breast in half but be careful not to cut all the way through. You are going to put the stuffing on one half and pull the other half over it when the chicken has been cooked.
3. Grease a casserole or baking pan.
4. Place the 2 cut-open chicken breasts in the dish/pan and place them in the oven.
5. Bake for approximately 25 to 30 minutes, turning the chicken over halfway through baking.
6. When there are 15 minutes left for the cooking of the chicken, start preparation on the filling and the sauce.
7. In a saucepan or microwaveable bowl, place the halved asparagus spears and mushrooms.

8. Add a dash of black pepper and crushed garlic.

9. If you are cooking on the stove, heat the ingredients until the butter has melted. The asparagus and mushrooms should be soft but still slightly firm.

10. Drain off excess butter.

11. When the chicken is cooked, remove it from the oven.

12. Add the cooked mushrooms and asparagus to the one-half of each of the chicken breasts.

13. Crumble goat cheese over the mushroom and asparagus filling.

14. Place half of the chicken breast without the filling over the top of the mixture.

15. Put the stuffed chicken breasts back into the oven and back for another 5 to 8 minutes, or until the goat cheese has melted.

16. While the chicken is baking, in a mixing bowl, mix together the mayonnaise and mustard powder.

17. When the chicken breasts are done, remove them from the oven.

18. Serve them on a dinner plate, topped with a dollop of mustard mayonnaise sauce, a dash of cayenne pepper, and a sprinkling of freshly chopped dill.

Chapter 12: Low-Carb Recipes for the Sweet Tooth

Here are 7 easy-to-make low-carb desserts or baked goods.

Please note that the nutritional information is per serving and that the carbohydrates reflect the **net carbs** and **not** the total carbs.

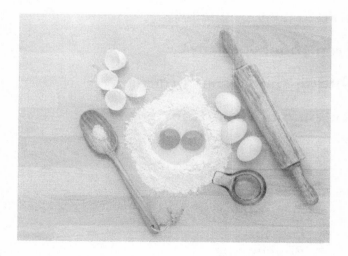

Recipe 22 — Bite-Sized Salted Caramel No-Bake Cheesecake Blocks

This delicious low-carb treat has under 1 g of net carbs per bite-sized block..

The recipe is suitable for Phase 2 to Phase 4.

Serving Size: 9 bite-sized blocks

Time: 1 hour 45 minutes

Prep Time: 15 minutes

Setting Time: 1 hour 30 minutes

Nutritional Facts/Info:

- Calories 66
- Net Carbs 0.9 g
- Fiber 3.1 g
- Sugars 0.3 g
- Fat 6.3 g
- Protein 1.9 g

Ingredients:

- ¼ cup macadamia nuts — crushed/bits
- ¼ tsp xanthan gum
- ¼ cup whey protein — unflavored or vanilla flavor can be used

- 3 tsp Stevia — sugar form and not the liquid
- 2 pinches of salt — up to ¼ tsp can be used
- 3 oz cream cheese
- ¼ cream — heavy
- 2 tsp caramel syrup — sugar-free
- ½ tsp vanilla extract

Directions:

1. Use a freezer-safe tray, approximately 7" w x 1.5" l x 1.5" deep.
2. Cut a piece of parchment paper big enough to cover the base and sides of the dish.
3. Place the parchment paper into the dish and put it to one side.
4. You can use an ice cube tray (lightly grease it) or freezer-safe silicone mold.
5. Whisk together the cream cheese, vanilla extract, 1 pinch of salt, and caramel syrup in a large mixing bowl.
6. Add the macadamia nuts, mixing them thoroughly into the mixture.
7. In another mixing bowl, mix the whey protein powder and cream until the mixture is smooth.
8. Fold the whey protein and cream mixture into the cream cheese mix, blend the mixture in a blender until smooth.
9. Add the xanthan gum and blend the mixture for another minute.

10. Pour the mixture into the freezer-safe dish.
11. Top with a light dash of salt.
12. Cover the mixture with plastic wrap.
13. Place the mixture in the freezer to set for 1 hour 30 minutes.
14. When the mixture has set, remove it from the freezer and cut into squares approximately 1-inch wide x ½-inch long.

Recipe 23 — Creamy Chocolate and Avocado Pudding

If you love chocolate pudding, you are going to love these low-carb chocolate and avocado pudding cups.

The recipe is suitable for Phase 2 to Phase 4.

Serving Size: 2

Time: 1 hour 15 minutes

Prep Time: 15 minutes

Setting Time: 1 hour

Nutritional Facts/Info:

- Calories 175
- Net Carbs 7 g
- Fiber 18.2 g
- Sugars 1.3 g
- Fat 7.2 g
- Protein 15.8 g

Ingredients:

- 2 tbsp mashed avocado
- 3 tbsp whey protein powder — vanilla or unflavored

- 2 tsp Stevia or sweetener of your choice from the approved food list
- ¾ tsp xanthan gum
- ½ tbsp cacao powder — unsweetened
- ½ tsp vanilla extract

Directions:

1. In a mixing bowl, blend together the avocado, cream, and whey protein powder until smooth.
2. Add the cacao powder, vanilla, xanthan gum, and Stevia.
3. Blend the mixture together until smooth and creamy.
4. Divide the mixture into 2 fridge safe small pudding bowls or cups.
5. Cover each bowl with plastic wrap.
6. Place the bowls in the refrigerator for 1 hour to set before serving.

Recipe 24 — *Spicy Dark Chocolate Chip Vanilla Cheesecake Pudding Cups*

This is a quick and easy to make vanilla cheesecake pudding. It has a rich warm flavor of allspice blended with the unique flavor of dark chocolate chips.

The recipe is suitable for Phase 1 to Phase 4.

Serving Size: 3

Time: 1 hour and 35 minutes

Prep Time: 15 minutes

Setting Time: 1 hour and 20 minutes

Nutritional Facts/Info:

- Calories 179
- Net Carbs 3.1 g
- Fiber 0.4 g
- Sugars 1.5 g
- Fat 18.3 g
- Protein 2.6 g

Ingredients:

- 1 tbsp dark chocolate nibs — sugar-free
- 3 oz cream cheese

- 3 tbsp cream — heavy
- ½ tbsp sour cream
- 1 ½ tbsp Stevia — powder/sugar and not the liquid
- ½ tsp allspice
- ½ tsp vanilla extract

Directions:

1. Place 3 pudding cups or small bowls into the freezer before you start to bake.
2. In a mixing bowl, blend together 1 tbsp Stevia, the sour cream, cream, cheese, and all-spice.
3. Blend together on medium until the mixture is thick and smooth.
4. Add the vanilla extract and chocolate chips; mix well.
5. In another mixing bowl, blend the heavy cream and ½ tbsp of Stevia until the cream thickens and forms soft peaks.
6. Fold the thickened cream into the sour cream and cream cheese mixture until it is well mixed together.
7. Using the iced pudding bowls from the freezer, spoon the mixture evenly into the 3 pudding bowls.
8. Cover each one with plastic wrap.
9. Place them in the refrigerator for 2 hours to set before serving.

Recipe 25 — Berry Cherry Ice Pops

These flavored fruit and berry pops are quick and easy to make. They will help to stave off your sweet tooth, they are refreshing, and a nice quick summer snack.

The recipe is suitable for Phase 2 to Phase 4.

Serving Size: 6 ice pops

Time: 2 hours 10 minutes to 4 hours 10 minutes

Prep Time: 10 minutes

Setting Time: 2 to 4 hours

Nutritional Facts/Info:

- Calories 11
- Net Carbs 1.8 g
- Fiber 1 g
- Sugars 1.6 g
- Fat 0.1 g
- Protein 0.2 g

Ingredients:

- ¼ cup blackberries — fresh or unsweetened frozen

- ¼ cup raspberries — fresh or unsweetened frozen
- ¼ cup blueberries — fresh or unsweetened frozen
- ¼ cup strawberries — fresh or unsweetened frozen
- 4 tbsp cherry syrup — sugar-free (Atkins or Da Vinci)
- 1 tsp lemon zest
- 1 tsp lime zest
- 1 cup of filtered water

Directions:

1. Blend the berries together with the filtered water.
2. Add the cherry syrup, lemon zest, and lime zest.
3. Blend for 30 seconds.
4. You can add another tbsp of cherry syrup if you feel it necessary.
5. Pour into 6 ice pop molds.
6. Place in the freezer for 2 to 4 hours or until completely set.

Recipe 26 — Refreshing Caramel Fruit and Berry Salad

This fruit salad makes a nice addition to a meal for Phase 3 and Phase 4. You can use it as a meal or halve it for a snack in Phase 2.

The recipe is suitable for Phase 2 to Phase 4.

Serving Size: 1

Time: 15 minutes

Prep Time: 15 minutes

Cook Time: N/A

Nutritional Facts/Info:

- Calories 151
- Net Carbs 8.1 g
- Fiber 2.4 g
- Sugars 7.3 g
- Fat 11.9 g
- Protein 1 g

Ingredients:

- 1 tbsp blackberries — fresh or unsweetened frozen

- 1 tbsp raspberries — fresh or unsweetened frozen
- 1 tbsp blueberries — fresh or unsweetened frozen
- ¼ cup honeydew melon — balls
- 1 tsp mint leaves — fresh and shredded
- 2 mint leaves — fresh
- 2 tbsp cream — heavy
- 2 tsp sour cream
- 1 tbsp caramel syrup — sugar-free (Da Vinci) optional
- 1 tsp Stevia or sweetener of your choice

Directions:

1. Place the berries, shredded mint, and honeydew melon in a bowl.
2. Place the bowl in the freezer for 10 minutes.
3. In a mixing bowl, blend the heavy cream together with the Stevia until the cream forms soft peaks.
4. Fold in the sour and caramel syrup.
5. After 10 minutes, remove the fruit and berries from the freezer.
6. Top with cream mixture.
7. Garnish with the two mint leaves and enjoy.

Recipe 27 — Nutty Crust Pumpkin Pie

This pie can be enjoyed in Phase 3.

The recipe is suitable for Phase 3 to Phase 4.

Serving Size: 8 slices

Time: 65 minutes

Prep Time: 15 minutes

Cook Time: 50 minutes

Nutritional Facts/Info:

- Calories 258
- Net Carbs 6.5 g
- Fiber 2.4 g
- Sugars 4.8 g
- Fat 23.8 g
- Protein 3.5 g

Ingredients:

- 2 eggs — large and at room temperature
- 2 cups walnuts — ground
- 1 ½ cups cream — heavy
- 2 cups pumpkin, canned, without salt
- ¼ cup butter — unsalted and melted
- 1 tsp allspice

- ½ tsp pumpkin spice
- ½ cup Stevia or sweetener of your choice from the approved food list
- 2 tsp Stevia (for the walnut base)
- dash of salt

Directions:

1. Preheat the oven to 325° F.
2. Combine the ground walnuts, melted butter, and 2 tsp of Stevia in a mixing bowl.
3. Lightly grease a 9-inch pie dish.
4. Firmly press the nut mixture into the pie dish to form a pie crust shell.
5. Place in the oven and bake for 10 minutes or until the crust turns golden brown. Be careful not to burn it.
6. While the pie crust is baking, prepare the filling.
7. Whisk together ½ cup of Stevia or sugar substitute, allspice, pumpkin spice, canned pumpkin, and add a dash of salt.
8. In another mixing bowl, mix the heavy cream until it forms soft firm peaks.
9. Fold the cream into the pumpkin mixture.
10. Place plastic wrap over it and place it in the fridge while the pie crust cools.
11. Remove the walnut crust pie shell from the oven and allow it to cool for 5 to 10 minutes.
12. Increase the heat of the oven to 375° F.

13. When the pie crust has cooled, take the pumpkin mixture out of the refrigerator and scoop it into the pie crust.
14. Distribute the mixture evenly.
15. Place the pie in the oven and bake for 30 to 40 minutes.
16. The middle of the pie should be nice and wobbly.
17. Cut into 6 pieces and serve.

Recipe 28 — Peppermint Chocolate Mousse

This minty chocolate mousse can be enjoyed from Phase 1.

The recipe is suitable for Phase 1 to Phase 4.

Serving Size: 3

Time: 1 hour and 15 minutes

Prep Time: 15 minutes

Setting Time: 1 hour

Nutritional Facts/Info:

- Calories 268
- Net Carbs 6.1g
- Fiber 0.9 g
- Sugars 6.3 g
- Fat 22.5 g
- Protein 8.5 g

Ingredients:

- 1 ½ scoop of whey protein — vanilla flavor
- 1 tsp cocoa powder — raw organic unsweetened
- 1 cups of cream — heavy
- 6 fresh mint leaves

- 1 tbsp Stevia or sweetener of your choice from the approved foods list
- ¼ tsp mint extract

Directions:

1. Place 3 pudding bowls in the freezer for 10 minutes.
2. Shred 4 of the fresh mint leaves and put the remaining two aside.
3. In a blender, beat the cream into soft stiff peaks.
4. Fold in the whey protein powder, cocoa powder, Stevia, shredded mint leaves, and peppermint extract.
5. Beat the ingredients until thick.
6. Remove the bowls from the freezer.
7. Scoop the mousse evenly into the 3 dessert bowls.
8. Cover each bowl with plastic wrap and place in the refrigerator.
9. Allow the mousse to set for at least 1 hour.
10. Remove from the refrigerator when the mousse has set and enjoy.

Chapter 13: Delicious Low-Carb Smoothies and Beverages

Here are 7 easy-to-make low-carb smoothies.

Please note that the nutritional information is per serving and that the carbohydrates reflect the **net carbs** and **not** the total carbs.

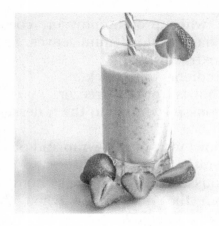

Recipe 29 — Peanut Butter Smoothie

Anyone who loves peanut butter is probably going to miss the peanut butter sandwiches as you are not able to eat bread, especially during the first few phases of the diet. This smoothie will satisfy both your hunger pangs and peanut butter cravings.

If you like eating peanut butter and celery, you can add 1 medium-sized chopped celery stalk to the recipe (0.2 net carbs).

You can use ¼ cup of coconut milk (2 g net carbs) instead of almond milk (0.3 g net carbs).

The recipe is suitable for Phase 1 to Phase 4.

Serving Size: 1

Time: 10 minutes

Prep Time: 10 minutes

Cook Time: N/A

Nutritional Facts/Info:

- Calories 292
- Net Carbs 6.1 g
- Fiber 3.4g
- Sugars 2.9 g

- Fat 21.4 g
- Protein 17.6 g

Ingredients:

- ½ cup of filtered water
- ½ cup almond milk — unsweetened, always choose the organic option if possible
- ½ tablespoon cocoa powder — unsweetened, the organic one is preferable
- 1 scoop whey protein powder — vanilla or chocolate flavor
- 2 tbsp peanut butter — smooth with no added sugar or salt
- 1 tsp/packet of Stevia sweetener or your preferred choice from the approved foods list
- ½ tsp vanilla extract
- ¼ tsp nutmeg

Directions:

1. In a blender or smoothie mixer, add the coconut milk, whey protein powder, water, and cocoa powder.
2. Blend together thoroughly.
3. Add peanut butter, vanilla, nutmeg, and Stevia.
4. Blend ingredients together thoroughly.
5. Pour into a glass or a sealed drinking flask/container.

Recipe 30 — Raspberry Coconut Zinger Smoothie

This smoothie comes with a bit of a bite as you add cayenne pepper and ginger.

You can use ¼ cup of coconut milk instead of ¼ almond milk; coconut milk is a lot higher in net carbs than almond milk.

The recipe is suitable for Phase 2 up to Phase 4.

Serving Size: 1

Time: 10 minutes

Prep Time: 10 minutes

Cook Time: N/A

Nutritional Facts/Info:

- Calories 189
- Net Carbs 6.1 g
- Fiber 4.5 g
- Sugars 3 g
- Fat 9 g
- Protein 19.6 g

Ingredients:

- 2 tbsp raspberries — fresh if possible, for frozen they must be unsweetened
- 1 tbsp shaved coconut — unsweetened
- ½ cup of filtered water
- ¼ cup almond milk — unsweetened and if possible look for organic
- 1 scoop protein whey powder — vanilla flavored
- ½ tsp cinnamon
- ½ tsp ground ginger
- ¼ tsp cayenne pepper

Directions:

1. Add all the ingredients into a blender or smoothie mixer.
2. Blend together thoroughly.
3. Pour into a glass or into a sealed drinking flask/container.

Recipe 31 — Blackberry Pecan Pie Smoothie

You can use ½ cup of coconut milk instead of ½ cup almond milk; remember to watch the net carbs as coconut milk is higher in carbs.

The recipe is suitable for Phase 2 to Phase 4.

Serving Size: 1

Time: 10 minutes

Prep Time: 10 minutes

Cook Time: N/A

Nutritional Facts/Info:

- Calories 164
- Net Carbs 4.9 g
- Fiber 3 g
- Sugars 2 g
- Fat 3.2 g
- Protein 8.6 g

Ingredients:

- 10 pecans
- 2 tbsp blackberries — fresh if possible, or unsweetened frozen
- ½ cup of filtered water

- ½ cup almond milk — unsweetened
- 1 scoop of whey protein powder — chocolate
- 2 tsp Stevia sweetener or a sweetener of your choice
- 3 tsp sugar-free maple syrup

Directions:

1. Add all the ingredients into a blender or smoothie mixer.
2. Blend together thoroughly.
3. Pour into a glass or into a sealed drinking flask/container.

Recipe 32 — *Chocolate, Mint, and Avocado Smoothie*

This smoothie can be enjoyed as a snack or a meal replacement.

You can add an optional 1 tsp of fresh basil to give it a unique flavor. You can also add a dash of cayenne pepper to get your metabolism going in the morning and give you some zing.

You can use 1 cup almond milk instead of 1 cup of coconut milk; you will need to adjust the net carb amount as coconut milk is higher in carbs than almond milk.

The recipe is suitable for Phase 1 to Phase 4.

Serving Size: 1

Time: 10 minutes

Prep Time: 10 minutes

Cook Time: N/A

Nutritional Facts/Info:

- Calories 209
- Net Carbs 5.7 g
- Fiber 4.6 g

- Sugars 1.7 g
- Fat 13.3 g
- Protein 14.2 g

Ingredients:

- ¼ avocado
- 1 tbsp (½ scoop) whey protein powder — chocolate
- 1 tsp fresh mint
- ¼ glass of filtered water
- ¼ cup coconut milk, unsweetened
- ¼ tsp vanilla extract
- ½ cinnamon

Directions:

1. Cut the avocado into cubes
2. In a blender, mix together all the ingredients.
3. Pour into a glass and enjoy it.

Recipe 33 — *Ginger, Cranberry, Cucumber, and Mint Fizz*

This is a nice refreshing drink to top up with during a meal or after a workout.

Enjoy this drink over a glass of crushed ice after a long hot day in the sun.

The recipe is suitable for Phase 1 to Phase 4.

Serving Size: 1

Time: 10 minutes

Prep Time: 10 minutes

Cook Time: N/A

Nutritional Facts/Info:

- Calories 20
- Net Carbs 2.1 g
- Fiber 0.7 g
- Sugars 0.5 g
- Fat 1.2 g
- Protein 0.4 g

Ingredients:

- 1 tbsp cranberries
- 2 tbsp cucumber — finely chopped

- 1 tsp ginger — fresh, grated
- 1 tbsp mint — fresh shredded
- 1 cup club soda
- 1 tsp Stevia or sweetener of choice from the approved foods list.

Directions:

1. Add all the ingredients into a blender.
2. Blend together thoroughly.
3. Pour into a glass and enjoy it.

Recipe 34 — Lemon and Lime Raspberry Watermelon Fizz

This drink can be enjoyed both fizzy and still by replacing the club soda with still water. Enjoy this drink over a few blocks of ice in the summer.

The recipe is suitable for Phase 2 to Phase 4.

Serving Size: 1

Time: 10 minutes

Prep Time: 10 minutes

Cook Time: N/A

Nutritional Facts/Info:

- Calories 32
- Net Carbs 6.8 g
- Fiber 2.8 g
- Sugars 3.2 g
- Fat 0.3 g
- Protein 0.8 g

Ingredients:

- ½ lime — peeled, remove pips, and chop into small chunks

- ½ lemon — peeled, remove pips, and chop into small chunks
- 2 tbsp watermelon — remove the rind, remove pips, and cut into cubes
- 2 tbsp raspberries — fresh, or unsweetened frozen
- 2 tsp Stevia or sweetener of your choice from the approved foods list.

Directions:

1. Add all the ingredients into a blender.
2. Blend together thoroughly.
3. Pour into a glass and enjoy it.

Recipe 35 — Salted Caramel Iced Coffee

If you have a sweet tooth, you can substitute one of your meals for this decadent low-carb smoothie.

You can swap the almond milk out for coconut milk if you want to; just remember to re-calculate the net carbs for the recipe.

The recipe is suitable for Phase 1 to Phase 4.

Serving Size: 1

Time: 10 minutes

Prep Time: 10 minutes

Cook Time: N/A

Nutritional Facts/Info:

- Calories 165
- Net Carbs 3.1 g
- Fiber 1 g
- Sugars 0.1 g
- Fat 4.9 g
- Protein 23.3 g

Ingredients:

- 1 scoop whey protein — chocolate flavor
- 2 tbsp cream cheese — fat-free
- 1 cup almond milk — unsweetened, organic if possible
- 2 tsp caramel syrup — sugar-free
- ½ tsp salt (you can add up to 1 tsp if desired)
- 1 tsp fine coffee powder — decaffeinated is the best choice
- ¼ cup crushed ice

Directions:

1. Add all the ingredients, except for the crushed ice, into a blender or smoothie mixer.
2. Blend together thoroughly.
3. Pour the crushed ice into a glass.
4. Pour the smoothie over the crushed ice and enjoy it.

Chapter 14: Additional Resources for Continued Success on the Atkins Diet

The Atkins website has a whole host of online resources that includes articles, tips, tricks, recipes, and products.

You can find additional Atkins resources, recipes, and products online. I have highlighted some of the most useful pages on the site for you below.

About the Atkins Diet and the History

To learn more about the Atkins Diet, the history, and why a low-carb diet promotes weight loss, the following link will give you access to the "Our Story" page on the Atkins Website:

https://www.atkins.com/our-mission

Articles, Blogs, and Helpful Information

For articles, references, success stories, and more information on the Atkins Diet, the following link will take you to the Atkins blog page.

https://www.atkins.com/how-it-works/atkins-blogs

Atkins Healthcare Professional Portal

The Atkins Healthcare Professional Portal is mainly accessed by healthcare professionals but you can find some information about the science behind the diet. You can also find some useful and informative articles. You can access the portal from the following link:

http://www.atkins-hcp.com/

Products

Atkins offers a lot of great low-carb nutritious and delicious products. These products include:

- Atkins bars
- Atkins Shakes
- Atkins Treats
- Atkins Frozen Food & Meals

The snack, treats, and shakes are a great way to stave off your sweet tooth and they can be used in various recipes that Atkins provides.

Another great product from Atkins is their frozen foods and meals. They are great time savers and you know you are getting a good nutritious meal.

When you access the products page, Atkins has a handy nearest store finder where you type in your zip code and it will direct you to the nearest stockist of Atkins products.

You can access the Atkins products page from the following link:

https://www.atkins.com/products

Recipes

The Atkins website is filled with low-carb recipes that have a convenient search facility that lets you search by recipe phase, meal type, or recipe name.

Each recipe will specify what phase the recipe is suited for and comes with a nutrition table. You can access the Atkins recipes page by following the link below:

https://www.atkins.com/recipes

Success Stories

You can read some heartwarming and encouraging Atkins Diet success stories at the following link:

https://www.atkins.com/success-stories

Leave a 1-Click Review!

Customer Reviews

⭐⭐⭐⭐⭐ 2
5.0 out of 5 stars ▾

5 star	████████	100%
4 star		0%
3 star		0%
2 star		0%
1 star		0%

See all verified purchase reviews ›

Share your thoughts with other customers

Write a customer review ⬅

I would be incredibly thankful if you could take just 60 seconds to write a brief review on Amazon, even if it's just a few sentences!

>> Scan with your camera to leave a quick review:

Conclusion

The Atkins Diet is not just a diet but a way of life. If you are serious about losing weight, getting healthy, and keeping the weight off, you need it to become your new lifestyle. When you start the diet, start thinking of the Atkins Diet as a lifetime commitment to a healthier, happier, and trimmer you. It may start off as a diet but it does not stop after the initial two to four weeks as it unfolds into a healthy eating plan.

Phase 1, the Inductions Phase, may seem pretty tough at first glance, but as you get into it, you will find there is a large variety of everyday foods to choose from. Play around with different recipes you find and make your own. Break out of your current comfort zone and let your taste buds expand their culinary horizons. A diet does not have to be boring; find the color and bring the choices you do have to life.

Phase 2 is the Continued Weight Loss Phase, which ups your carbs a bit and throws in some more foods you can eat. By the time you get to this phase, you will already be adding those carbs up in your head and designing your own low-carb dishes. Even if you are not a great cook, check out the easy-to-follow recipes included in this book and reinvent them.

Phase 3 is the Pre-Maintenance Phase. At this stage, you're at the border of reaching your goal weight. You are getting ready to step out of the diet mode into maintenance mode. This is the phase where you will start to learn how to manage your weight and food so you can confidently progress into the next stage.

Phase 4 is the Maintenance or Lifestyle Phase. This is the stage where you are ready to leave the Atkins Diet nest and take your first solo flight into the Atkins Lifestyle. Join various Atkins Diet support groups and newsletters. Keeping up with the dieting and eating trends is an important part of changing to a healthier lifestyle. There are always new developments and foods that all help you maintain your new lifestyle.

Exercise complements your weight loss regimen and will help to firm and tone your body. Exercise also offers health benefits and boosts your self-confidence. Just don't overdo the exercise.

Use the meal plans and acceptable food lists from the chapters above to make quick and easy grocery lists. Fill up on water or at least have a low-carb snack before you go do your grocery shopping to stop cravings and filling up on junk food high in carbs.

Don't get despondent if you have off-days or slip-ups; take them as they come, forgive yourself for them, and move on. Most importantly, remember not to give up, keep pushing through. Nothing is ever easy to begin with, but the end result is well worth the effort.

If you have made it to the end of the book and have started your Atkins lifestyle journey, well done.

As I love to hear from my readers, please leave a review and let me know how you enjoyed the book.

Enjoy the new healthier and slimmer you!

SPECIAL BONUS!

Want This Bonus book for FREE?

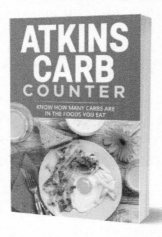

Get FREE unlimited access to it and all of my new books by joining the Fan Base!

SCAN W/ YOUR CAMERA TO JOIN!

References

Atkins for Vegans. (n.d.). Atkins. https://www.atkins-hcp.com/atkins-resources/research/atkins-for-vegans-1

Atkins for Veggies. (n.d.). Atkins. https://uk.atkins.com/blog/atkins-for-veggies/

Butler, N. (2020, January 30). *Atkins diet: What is it, and should I try it?* Medical News Today. https://www.medicalnewstoday.com/articles/7379

Carbohydrates. (n.d.). Cleveland Clinic. https://my.clevelandclinic.org/health/articles/15416-carbohydrates

Coyle, D. (2018, October 03). *Starchy vs Non-Starchy Vegetables: Food Lists and Nutrition Facts.* Healthline. https://www.healthline.com/nutrition/starchy-vs-

Gardner, C., Klazand, A., & Alhassan, S. (200, March 7). *Comparison of the Atkins, Zone, Ornish, and LEARN Diets for Change in Weight and Related Risk Factors Among Overweight Premenopausal Women The A*

TO Z Weight Loss Study: A Randomized Trial. JAMA Network. https://jamanetwork.com/journals/jama/fullarticle/205916

How It Works. (n.d.). Atkins. https://www.atkins.com/how-it-works

Low Carb Diet Rules of Induction. (n.d.). Atkins. https://www.atkins.com/how-it-works/library/articles/the-rules-of-induction

Mandes, T. (2014, December 09). *The Difference Between Processed and Refined Foods.* Trisha Mandes. http://www.trishamandes.com/blog/2014/12/8/the-difference-between-processed-and-refined-foods

Metcalfe, R. (2019, March 20). *Even light physical activity has health benefits – new research.* The Conversation. https://theconversation.com/even-light-physical-activity-has-health-benefits-new-research-113700

Nutrition 101. (n.d.). Build Healthy Kids. http://www.buildhealthykids.com/basics.html

Scott, J. (2020, September 12). *What You Can Drink on the Atkins Diet*. Verywell Fit. https://www.verywellfit.com/what-you-can-drink-during-induction-on-the-atkins-diet-3496207#:

Warburton, D., Nicol, C., & Bredin, S. (2006, March 14). *Health benefits of physical activity: the evidence*. NCBI. https://www.ncbi.nlm.nih.gov/pmc/articles/PMC1402378/

What are Net Carbs? How to Calculate Net Carbs. (n.d.). Atkins. https://www.atkins.com/how-it-works/library/articles/what-are-net-carbs

Image References

Congerdesign. (2017, November 17). *Pumpkin Soup* [Photograph]. Pixabay. https://pixabay.com/photos/pumpkin-soup-soup-2972858/

Free-Photos. (2015, September 11). *Dinner* [Photograph]. https://pixabay.com/photos/meal-food-dinner-lunch-restaurant-918639/

J. (2017, December 3). *Sprouts, avocado, berries, lettuce, and nut board* [Photograph]. https://pixabay.com/photos/broccoli-sprouts-super-food-1977732/

Kerdkanno, S. (2015, August 28). *Baking* [Photograph]. https://pixabay.com/photos/background-baker-baking-cooking-906135/

Kulesza, M. (2018, May 15). *Don't Give Up* [Photograph]. https://pixabay.com/photos/don-t-give-up-motivation-3403779/

PhotoMix-Company. (2016, May 27). *Strawberry Smoothie* [Photograph].

https://pixabay.com/photos/strawberry-smoothie-kefir-the-drink-1418212/

Reche, D. (2020, June 22). *Walking/Running* [Photograph]. https://pixabay.com/photos/running-sport-race-athlete-hall-4782721/

StockSnap. (2017, July 31). *Yoga/Pilates* [Photograph]. https://pixabay.com/photos/people-woman-yoga-meditation-2562357/

Tuso, J. (n.d.). *Nutritional Update for Physicians: Plant-Based Diets.* NCBI. https://www.ncbi.nlm.nih.gov/pmc/article s/PMC3662288/

Vegan Liftz. (2019, May 27). *Meal Plan* [Photograph]. https://pixabay.com/photos/meal-plan-diet-plan-eating-healthy-4232109/

Wellington, J. (2018, March 11). *Basket of brown eggs.* https://pixabay.com/photos/brown-eggs-breakfast-nutrition-food-3217675/